Emergencies in Eyecare

Emergencies in Eyecare

Leslie Hargis-Greenshields, COMT

Linda Sims, COT

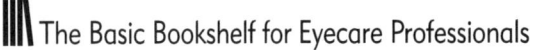
The Basic Bookshelf for Eyecare Professionals

Series Editors: Janice K. Ledford, COMT • Ken Daniels, OD • Robert Campbell, MD

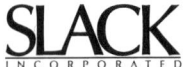 6900 Grove Road, Thorofare, NJ 08086

Publisher: John H. Bond
Editorial Director: Amy E. Drummond
Assistant Editor: Lauren E. Biddle

Copyright © 1999 by SLACK Incorporated

All rights reserved. No part of this book may be reproduced, stored in a retrieval system or transmitted in any form or by any means, electronic, mechanical, photocopying, recording or otherwise, without written permission from the publisher, except for brief quotations embodied in critical articles and reviews.

Printed in the United States of America

Hargis-Greenshields, Leslie.
    Emergencies in eyecare/Leslie Hargis-Greenshields, Linda Sims.
        p. cm. -- (The basic bookshelf for eyecare professionals)
    Includes bibliographical references and index.
    ISBN 1-55642-354-3 (alk. paper)
    1. Ophthalmologic emergencies. I. Sims, Linda. II. Title. III. Series.
    [DNLM: 1. Eye Injuries. 2. Emergencies. 3. Eye Diseases. WW 525 H279e 1999]
    RE48.H34 1999
    617.7'025--dc21
    DNLM/DLC
    for Library of Congress   99-15135
                                                                                                  CIP

Published by: SLACK Incorporated
                  6900 Grove Road
                  Thorofare, NJ 08086-9447 USA
                  Telephone: 609-848-1000
                                856-848-1000
                  Fax: 609-853-5991
                        856-853-5991
                  World Wide Web: http://www.slackinc.com

Contact SLACK Incorporated for more information about other books in this field or about the availability of our books from distributors outside the United States.

Authorization to photocopy items for internal or personal use, or the internal or personal use of specific clients, is granted by SLACK Incorporated, provided that the appropriate fee is paid directly to Copyright Clearance Center, 222 Rosewood Drive, Danvers, MA 01923 USA, 978-750-8400. Prior to photocopying items for educational classroom use, please contact the CCC at the address above. Please reference Account Number 9106324 for SLACK Incorporated's Professional Book Division.

For further information on CCC, check CCC Online at the following address: http://www.copyright.com.

Last digit is print number: 10 9 8 7 6 5 4 3 2 1

Dedication

I would like to dedicate my portion of this project to my parents, Ed and Frances Hargis, who have been terrific references, as well as never-ending sources of support; to my husband, Mark, who has been extremely patient and supportive of all of my projects; and to my daughter, Kallie, who has been with me from the beginning (you are my reason!).

Leslie Hargis-Greenshields, COMT

I would like to dedicate this book to my parents, Bill and Elsie Sims, my sister, my brothers, and my aunt Katherine. They have been my source of strength, as well as the people who inadvertently provided that initial spark of interest that lead me into the field of ophthalmology.

Linda Sims, COT

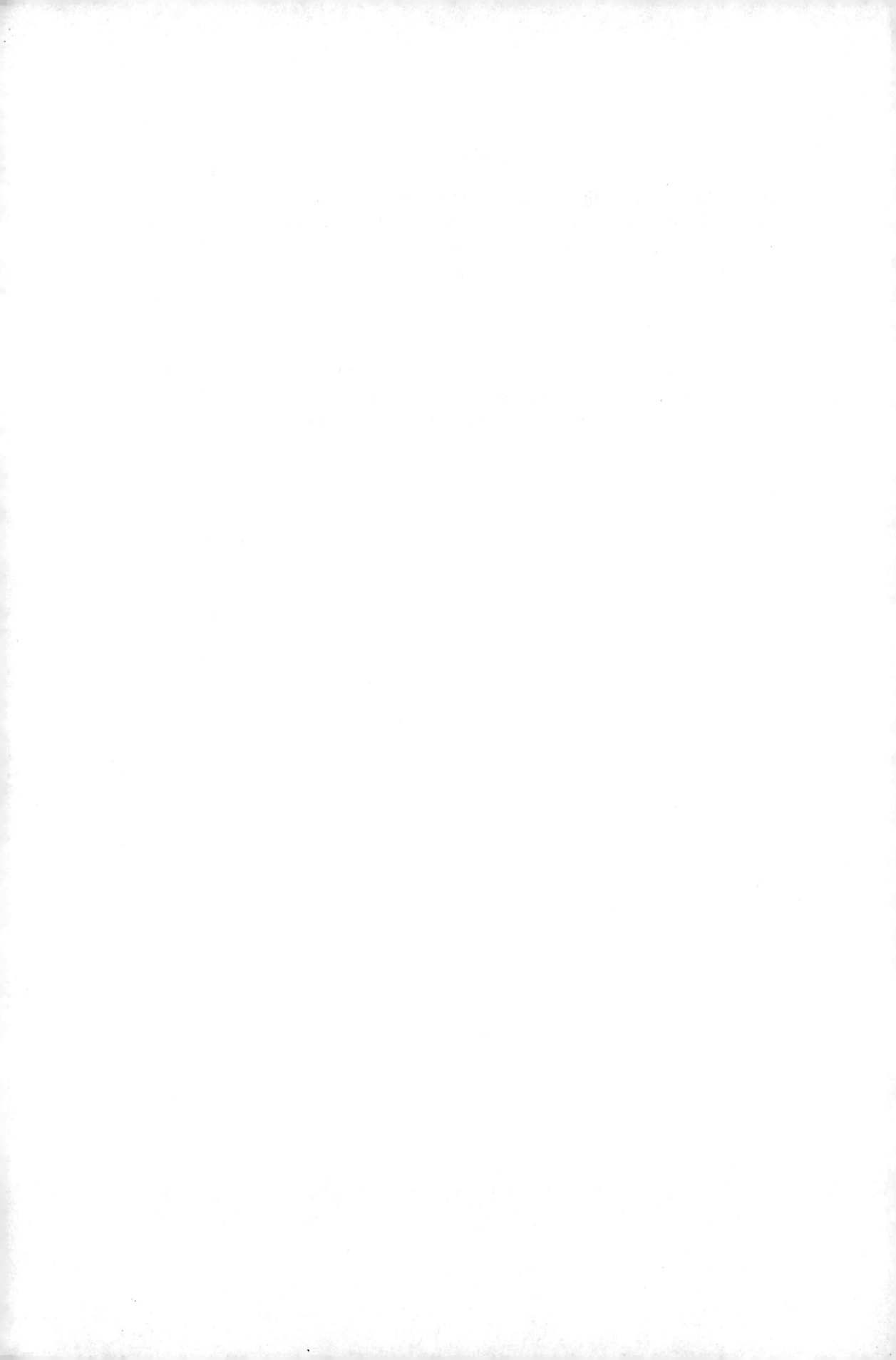

Contents

Dedications .... *v*
Acknowledgments .... *ix*
About The Authors .... *xi*
Introduction .... *xiii*
The Study Icons .... *xv*

Chapter 1. Triage 1
    Leslie Hargis-Greenshields, COMT

Chapter 2. Emergencies and Injuries of the Lids and Lacrimal System 11
    Linda Sims, COT

Chapter 3. Emergencies and Injuries of the Orbit 19
    Linda Sims, COT

Chapter 4. Emergencies and Injuries of the Conjunctiva, Sclera, and Cornea 25
    Linda Sims, COT

Chapter 5. Emergencies and Injuries of the Lens 45
    Leslie Hargis-Greenshields, COMT

Chapter 6. Glaucoma 53
    Leslie Hargis-Greenshields, COMT

Chapter 7. Emergencies and Injuries of the Uveal Tract 63
    Janice K. (Jan) Ledford, COMT

Chapter 8. Emergencies and Injuries of the Vitreous and Retina 71
    Linda Sims, COT

Chapter 9. The Red Eye 85
    Linda Sims, COT

Chapter 10. First Aid and Office Emergencies...105
    Linda Sims, COT

Chapter 11. Cardiopulmonary Resuscitation 117
    Leslie Hargis-Greenshields, COMT

Bibliography *139*
Index *143*

Acknowledgments

I would like to begin by thanking my father for giving me my first taste of ophthalmology. His kindness, compassion, and surgical skill will forever be a source of admiration.

I would like to acknowledge Drs. Michael Lins and Alan Sadowsky, whose practice will always be my measuring stick. Thank you for the opportunity and your friendship.

A big thank you to all my family. I am truly blessed.

To Paula Parker my role model and friend: thank you for your support.

To Jan Ledford, our editor, for her gentle encouragement: you are much appreciated.

And finally, to Linda Sims, who (as always) rises to the occasion and then surpasses all expectations. You are amazing.

Leslie Hargis-Greenshields, COMT

I would like to acknowledge those in the ophthalmic and optometric communities with whom I have had the pleasure of working through the years. I appreciate the support of these doctors, managers, and ophthalmic medical personnel, and the opportunities I have had to learn and grow.

I would also like to acknowledge Dr. Claude Miller and Dr. Robert Francis, the eye surgeons whom I was fortunate to know during critical times in my life. Thank you both for your expertise and skill.

A special thank you to my co-author, mentor and friend, Leslie Hargis-Greenshields, for believing in me. Thanks also to my editor, Jan Ledford, and my sister Bonnie, who have been amazingly patient and supportive throughout this project.

I truly appreciate all of you.

Linda Sims, COT

Editor's note: We would also like to thank the following people who were willing to pose for photographs: Jim Ledford, Connie Smith, Richard Echelman, Charles Kirby, Denise Queen, Heather Stamey, and John Hopkins.

About The Authors

Leslie Hargis-Greenshields, COMT

Leslie is a 1984 graduate of the St. Paul Ramsey School for Ophthalmic Technicians. Over the past 15 years she has worked in university settings as well as private clinics. Each opportunity has provided a new exposure in diagnostics, teaching, research, and administration.

Leslie has been very involved in teaching at both local and national levels. She is also a co-founder and partner of a consulting company, Ocular Training Concepts (OTC). This company provides training and educational opportunities in office settings and regional seminars for allied health personnel in the field of ophthalmology.

Leslie is currently the Director of Clinical Operations at TLC Northwest Eye Clinic in Seattle.

Linda Sims, COT

Linda Sims obtained her Bachelor of Arts degree in Psychology from Central Washington University in 1978. She was employed for many years as an optometric assistant/optician/office manager, which provided her with a solid knowledge base regarding eyeglasses, contact lenses, optics, and business operations. She joined the ophthalmic support staff of Group Health Cooperative in 1993, earning her certification at the assistant level and then at the technician level. She has been employed at Virginia Mason Medical Center since 1998. Linda has been active on the planning committees of the Washington Academy of Eye Physicians and Surgeon's Assistants annual continuing education program for 1997 and 1998.

Introduction

While many emergencies and urgent situations are described in this book, it is not possible to cover every situation that may arise. The best course of action for any emergency situation is to be prepared. Prepare through staff education. Have office procedures and protocols in place. Know where your emergency supplies are kept and how to use them. Know and post emergency aid phone numbers. Have periodic emergency preparedness reviews. Anything you can do to prepare ahead of time will save precious seconds when an emergency inevitably occurs.

The best we can do in this book is to present many emergent and urgent situations, with recommended protocol and a review of accepted treatment courses. However, remember that there may be an overlap in degree of urgency. A routine problem may border on the semi-urgent. What appears initially to be an urgent situation may in fact be emergent. Use your specific office protocol, your knowledge, and your common sense when dealing with an emergent situation. Always err on the side of caution. Your patients may be depending on you not only for their eyesight, but in some instances, for their lives.

Be prepared.

The Study Icons

The Basic Bookshelf for Eyecare Professionals is quality educational material designed for professionals in all branches of eyecare. Because so many of you want to expand your careers, we have made a special effort to include information needed for certification exams. When these study icons appear in the margin of a series book, it is your cue that the material next to the icon (which may be a paragraph or an entire section) is listed as a criteria item for a certification examination. Please use this key to identify the appropriate icon:

OptA	optometric assistant
OptT	optometric technician
OphA	ophthalmic assistant
OphT	ophthalmic technician*
OphMT	ophthalmic medical technologist*
LV	low vision subspecialty
Srg	ophthalmic surgical assisting subspecialty
CL	contact lens registry
Optn	opticianry
RA	retinal angiographer

*Because these icons apply to the entire text, they will not appear anywhere on the pages.

Chapter 1

Triage

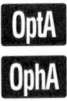

Leslie Hargis-Greenshields, COMT

KEY POINTS

- Triage is the screening of patients to determine the urgency of their situation.
- The purpose of triage is to ensure that patients with the most serious complaints are seen or referred promptly.
- Conditions may be rated as emergent, urgent, or elective.
- Each practice or clinic should set up protocols and procedures regarding triage specific to that practice.
- The anxiety of the patient also plays a key role in how soon he or she should be seen.

The military was the first to triage wounded patients on the battlefield. A five-tier rating system was used dependent upon the seriousness of the injury and the availability of treatment. Each situation was classified as:

- Dead or dying
- Life-threatening
- Urgent
- Delayed
- No injury

In eyecare we use a three-tier system and classify each situation as:

- Emergent (to be seen immediately)
- Urgent (to be seen same or next day)
- Elective (or routine exam within 1 to 2 weeks)

Phone and Office

Whether answering the phone or greeting a patient walking into the office, you are the primary contact between the patient and the physician (Figure 1-1). The patient expects to receive prompt, courteous, and reliable assistance. The physician expects you to accurately assess the seriousness of a situation and to take appropriate action. Set up a time with your doctor to determine specific policies regarding telephone and office triage. You will want to know the doctor's expectations of you in these situations.

Your role in triage is to first determine the patient's chief complaint. This can be accomplished by asking the patient to describe what kind of problems he or she is having. Next, assess the seriousness of the complaint by classifying the situation as emergent, urgent, or elective. It is important to follow protocol and procedures specific to your office.

If a patient describes a situation about which you are unsure, do not hesitate to ask the doctor for direction. The physician would rather have you ask questions than run the risk of delaying a patient who may need emergent attention. If you are having difficulty placing a specific complaint into one of the categories, it is best to err on the side of caution. Remember, your role is to determine the chief complaint, assess its seriousness, and follow procedures specific to your office.

Never give medical advice or diagnose possible problems, no matter how "simple" they seem. Even if you are sure of what the patient is describing, let his or her answers to your questions lead the doctor to a diagnosis, not you.

An important part of triage screening includes being calm, courteous, and reassuring. Courtesy is always a necessity. Smile when you answer the phone. This comes through in your voice and goes a long way in building the patient's confidence in your ability to assess his or her needs.

Not only are you assessing the medical needs of the patient, you are also evaluating his or her emotional needs as well. Listen to the patient, who often knows how serious the situation is. Remain calm and reassuring. This provides comfort to the patient in a stressful situation. Let the anxiety of the patient help to dictate when he or she should be seen. If a patient is extremely upset or anxious and is ready to crawl through the phone, it may be prudent to have him or her come into the office immediately, even if the situation does not constitute an emergency.

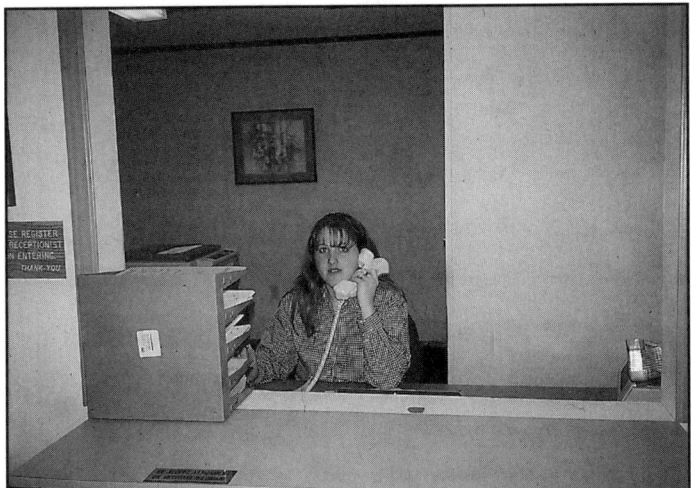

Figure 1-1. Triage often begins on the phone.

What the Patient Needs to Know

- We are trying to determine the urgency of your situation. We will have to ask you a series of questions.

- Some cases are more urgent than others. Sight-threatening problems are seen the same day.

- If you have a future appointment but your vision changes, you experience pain, or your symptoms become worse, do not hesitate to call us sooner.

- Broken glasses are not usually an emergency; however, please tell us if you are severely handicapped (ie, unable to drive) without them and have no spare pair.

History Taking in Emergency Situations

Using a screening form (Figure 1-2) when taking messages is helpful. It allows you to have a list of the most important questions to ask the patient and it provides a place to record the responses.

Basic History Questions

Your role is now that of a detective. You must find out as quickly and efficiently as possible how, what, where, and when an injury or problem happened (Figure 1-3). Ask the patient:
- What is the problem?
- When did the problem start? (In general, the more recent the onset of symptoms, the more urgent the situation.) Is it getting worse?
- Is the eye painful?
- Are there any vision changes?
- Has the eye been injured? How was it injured? When did the injury take place?

Ocular Training Concepts
Telephone Screening Form

Date _____ Time _____

Patient_____ DOB_____ Phone(H)_____(W)_____

ID#_____Person calling_____ Pt.Address_____

Next appt_____ Initials_____ Physician_____Location_____

CC(What is the Problem?)   OD   OS   OU

_____

_____

_____

When did it Start?_____ Onset: Sudden / Gradual   Getting Better/ Worse/ Stable

Has this occurred before?   Yes   No

Are there any vision changes?   Yes   No   Distance / Near / Both

Pain?   Yes   No   Redness?   Yes   No

Recent Eye Surgery?   Yes   No   Contact Lenses?   Yes   No

Other Symptoms?

_____

_____

Medications?

_____

Allergies?

_____

Assessment of patients desire to be seen.   High   Low

MD Instructions:

_____

_____

_____

Figure 1-2. Screening form.

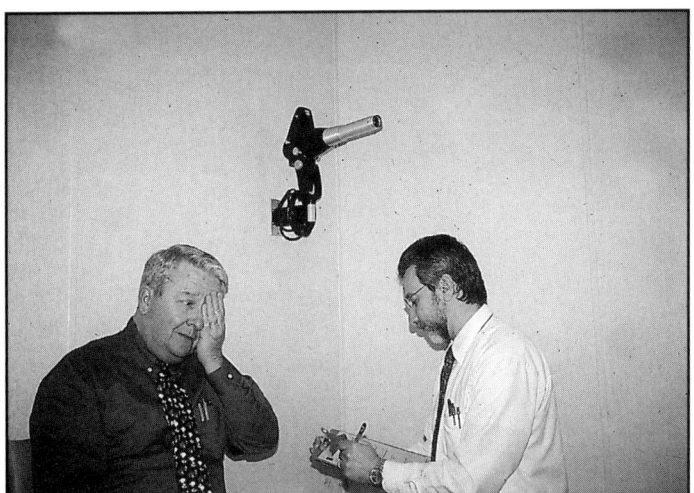

Figure 1-3. The patient history is also an opportunity for triage.

In addition, you should find out:
- Are there other eye problems? Any preexisting conditions?
- Is the patient monocular? (Keep in mind that a person with functional vision in only one eye is considered monocular.)
- Is the patient on any eye medications? Is this a glaucoma patient?
- Does the patient wear contact lenses?
- Is this a postoperative patient?

Additional information may be needed following irrigation of a chemical injury:
- The patient's visual acuity (when possible).
- The name or type of chemical involved. (Know how to reach your area's poison control agency to find a compound's chemical makeup.) Examples:
    Bleach—3% sodium hypochlorite—pH 1.0
    Toilet cleaner—sulfuric acid (80%)—pH 1.0
    Drain cleaner—sodium or potassium hydroxide—pH 14
    Ammonia—ammonium hydroxide (9%)—pH 12.5
    (The normal pH of the eye is roughly 7.4.)
- A summary of the accident, including details as to the extent of the exposure to the chemical. Examples:
    a. A large quantity splashed directly into the eye.
    b. Fumes from a chemical irritated the eye.
    c. A small amount of chemical transferred from the finger to the eye.

Emergent Category

Ophthalmic emergencies are those situations that require immediate action. If you determine that a patient has a medical emergency, advise him or her to come into the office immediately or to go to the nearest medical or emergency facility capable of treating ophthalmic problems. If the situation warrants, you may want to offer to call a cab or ambulance to help the patient. In eyecare we can break this category into more specific sections: emergent where treatment is required within minutes, and emergent where treatment is required within hours.

Treatment Within Minutes

There are three *true* ocular emergencies where treatment is required within minutes:

1. Chemical burns of the eye
2. Sudden loss of vision
3. Penetrating injuries of the eye

Chemical Burns of the Eye

Any patient who telephones the office to report a chemical in the eye should be instructed to irrigate the affected eye immediately by holding it open under gently running water for at least 15 to 20 minutes before coming to the office or proceeding to an emergency facility. Once the patient arrives in the office, chemical burns must be treated immediately by further irrigating the eye with large amounts of sterile saline solution or tap water. It is important that the assistant taking the initial call inform the back office staff and physician of the type of injury to make sure irrigation continues as soon as the patient arrives at the office. Chemical burns are discussed in more detail in Chapter 4.

Alkali burns tend to be the most destructive type of chemical injury. The severity of these burns is related to the fact that alkali becomes adherent to the corneal and conjunctival tissues and produces chemical reactions between its products and the tissue proteins. Several common alkaline products involved in chemical burns are ammonia (used in cleaning materials) and calcium hydroxide or lime (used in cements, mortars, and plasters).

Acid burns tend to be less caustic to the eye, but still require immediate irrigation both at the site of occurrence and at the physician's office. Acid injuries frequently result from exploding car batteries or laboratory test accidents, which may be complicated by the involvement of glass or other particles.

Organic solvents include kerosene, gasoline, alcohol, and cleaning fluids. Organic solvent injuries also require immediate irrigation both at the site and in the physician's office.

Sudden, Painless Loss of Vision

Any person describing a sudden, painless loss of vision should be suspected of having a central retinal artery occlusion (CRAO). CRAOs actually block the inflow of blood and oxygen to the central retina. They occur most often from an embolus or thrombus in persons with hypertension or atherosclerosis. Another cause is temporal arteritis or giant cell arteritis.

In any instance of a CRAO, the retina is completely without blood as long as the artery is occluded. The eye will go completely blind if immediate ophthalmic treatment is not initiated. The ophthalmologist may attempt to dislodge the occlusion by passing a sharp instrument into the anterior chamber. Aqueous fluid is allowed to escape or is removed with a needle, causing a sudden decrease in the intraocular pressure (IOP) which may restore blood flow to the central retinal artery. Other measures may be taken, such as ocular massage or breathing into a paper bag (which increases the levels of carbon dioxide and may induce retinal vasodilation).

Other conditions with the same symptoms of sudden, painless loss of vision include: vitreous hemorrhage, massive retinal detachment (RD), central retinal vein occlusion (CRVO), and retrobulbar neuritis. Treatment in these cases can be instituted within hours rather than minutes; however, anyone complaining of sudden, painless loss of vision should be treated as an emergency patient.

Penetrating Injuries of the Eye

Always suspect penetration of the globe when there are small lacerations of the lid due to high velocity missiles, injuries from wire, or accidents involving shattered glass. Rupture of the globe is always a serious injury that may result in blindness or even loss of the eyeball. Care must be taken not to press on the globe.

Treatment Within Hours

Other than the three *true* ocular emergencies, treatment of these emergent cases require examination to take place within hours:

- Acute ocular trauma, including blunt trauma, especially if accompanied by visual loss or visual abnormality
- Foreign body (FB) or corneal abrasion caused by an FB
- Recent onset of eye pain with or without redness
- Recent onset of flashing lights or floaters
- Pain or redness with contact lens usage
- Monocular patients with ocular complaints
- Postoperative patients with ocular complaints

Acute ocular trauma includes blunt trauma, such as a forceful blow to the eye from a fist or racquetball. There are numerous possible results, ranging from ecchymosis (bruising) to traumatic cataracts, RDs, and optic nerve injuries. Any acute trauma to the eye, especially if accompanied by visual abnormalities or loss, needs to be treated on an emergent basis.

FBs, or abrasions of the cornea caused by FBs, are the most frequent type of eye injury. These tend to be particularly painful and need to be seen the same day to remove the FB and treat the possible abrasion.

A recent onset of eye pain with or without redness is of concern due to the serious nature of the problems it suggests (see Chapter 9). Sharp stabbing pain usually indicates a corneal problem, while dull aches usually indicate a problem inside the eye. In either event, the patient complaining of a sudden onset of pain needs to see the eyecare specialist the same day.

A recent onset of floaters, spots, cobwebs, and flashing lights are often the precursor of an RD, vitreous detachment, or hemorrhage. A vitreous floater is a vitreous opacity that stimulates the retina by casting a shadow. Patients describe these shadows as spots, threads, particles, cobwebs, or flies. The spots move when the eye moves, and continue to move after the eye comes to rest. It is the sudden onset of floaters or the recent change of the appearance of floaters that is cause for the emergent concern.

Pain or redness in contact lens wearers could indicate infections or corneal ulcers. Because of the seriousness of these situations, the contact lens wearer that describes pain or redness of either eye should be told to remove the lens immediately and then seen in the office the same day.

Monocular patients are generally triaged using the emergent guidelines. Since they have functioning vision in only one eye, extra precautions should be taken.

Postoperative patients require preferential treatment when calling the office with problems. Unusual pain, redness, discharge, or swelling could indicate an infection. There could also be a reaction to the medications or sutures.

Urgent Category

Urgent situations require that the patient be seen within 24 to 48 hours after calling the eye-care specialist. Patients may report a variety of symptoms that need prompt attention. It may be difficult to distinguish an urgent situation from an emergency. If you have any questions, the safest course of action is to consult with the physician. When in doubt, err on the side of caution.

The following conditions fall into the urgent category:
- Recent onset of double vision
- Sudden onset of ptosis (a droopy lid)
- Photophobia (light sensitivity)
- Distorted vision for less than 2 weeks
- Eye pain for more than 48 hours but less than 1 week
- Colored halos around lights

Double vision is of urgent importance because it occurs as a result of disease within the brain, in the extraocular muscles (EOMs) themselves, or in the nerves going to the EOMs. Among the more serious conditions producing double vision are brain tumors, aneurysm, stroke, diabetes, and trauma (such as a blow-out fracture).

Weakness of the levator muscle results in lid droop, or ptosis. The significance of an acquired droopy lid (ie, cause has not been previously determined) holds the same urgent importance as double vision, since the symptom may be produced by the same serious conditions.

Photophobia is an unusual sensitivity to light and deserves urgent attention. This symptom usually accompanies a painful red eye stemming from conditions such as corneal inflammation and iritis. Aphakia and ocular albinism, as well as some medications, may also be accompanied by light sensitivity. Examples of such medications include penicillin, chloroquine, and acetazolamide.

Distorted vision for less than 2 weeks may be due to disorders of the media, retina, optic nerve, or brain, and should be considered urgent. The most common reason for distorted vision is a problem with the macula.

Eye pain for more than 48 hours but less than 1 week is a category that can cover a variety of conditions such as infections, allergies, and inflammations of the eye. The important point to remember is that this is not a sudden onset of eye pain, which would classify it as an emergency.

Colored halos or rings seen when viewing lights is an important sign of an impending angle-closure glaucoma attack. Other causes are corneal edema or infiltrates, foreign material in the tear film, and lens changes.

Elective Category

The elective problem often includes conditions that have been present for several weeks or more. These conditions usually do not pose an immediate threat to the patient's vision. However, if the patient is concerned or anxious, even though the medical condition is more routine, let the patient's anxiety help dictate how soon he or she should be seen. Do not hesitate to ask the physician for the answer to any question about which you are unsure. Always remind patients to contact the office if symptoms become worse, or if vision becomes impaired between appointments.

Conditions that fall into the elective category:
- Gradual visual loss for more than 3 weeks
- Headaches not accompanied by other symptoms
- Eye itching, tearing, or discharge, for more than 3 weeks
- Mild redness for more than 3 weeks not accompanied by other symptoms
- Masses on lids
- Broken glasses

Gradual visual loss in quiet eyes is frequently caused by uncorrected refractive errors. Other causes include cataracts and macular degeneration. The important point is that this loss of vision is gradual.

Headaches not accompanied by other symptoms are usually not caused from eye problems. However, to differentiate some of the more serious causes of headaches the patient should be asked about the quality of the headache (sharp stabbing pain or dull ache), location, duration, frequency, and details of the onset.

Itching, tearing, discharge, and redness for more than 3 weeks are most frequently caused by inflammation of the lids or conjunctiva (ie, chronic blepharitis, conjunctivitis, and allergic reactions like hay fever).

As long as no pain is involved and the vision is not affected, lid lesions should be treated as an elective problem. The most disconcerting aspect of the mass or lump on an eyelid is the cosmetic disfigurement of the face. The most common cause of lumps is a sweat gland infection known as hordeolum (stye). A second cause is a blocked meibomian gland, commonly called a chalazion.

Broken glasses can be a traumatic situation for the patient; however, it is typically not considered an emergent or urgent situation. Still, the person with a moderate to high refractive error may not be able to function without correction, so it is best to follow the protocol appropriate to your office to handle this situation.

Chapter 2

Emergencies and Injuries of the Lids and Lacrimal System

OphA

Linda Sims, COT

KEY POINTS

- The eyelids are the first source of protection for the eyes.
- Many lid infections and inflammations may be uncomfortable for the patient, but are usually not vision- or life-threatening.
- Carcinomas can invade lid tissues.
- Eyelid trauma is often accompanied by ocular trauma.
- Lid lacerations may be accompanied by a perforated globe.
- Chemical burns may affect the lids as well as the eye and need immediate, thorough rinsing.
- Thermal burns may be superficial or very deep, affecting the full thickness of the lid and surrounding structures.

Anatomy of the Lids and Lacrimal System

The eyelids provide protection to the anterior portions of the eye by shielding the eyes from injury, light, and tear evaporation. They also aid in distributing tear film with each blink.

The lids are made up of an outer layer of skin, a middle layer of muscle, a fibrous plate-like tissue called the tarsal plate (or tarsus, which gives the eyelids their shape), and the conjunctiva (an inner layer of mucous membrane tissue). The eyelid muscles include the orbicularis oculi that closes the eye when it contracts and the levator palpebrae superioris that raises the upper lid.

The conjunctiva begins as the palpebral conjunctiva, which makes up the inner lining of the lids, and continues on to become the bulbar conjunctiva, which covers the sclera to the limbus. The junction of the palpebral and bulbar conjunctiva is called the fornix.

The lid margins contain the eyelash follicles, the eyelashes (cilia), and the meibomian glands.

The opening between the eyelids is known as the palpebral fissure. The nasal junction of the upper and lower lids is called the medial canthus. The temporal junction of the lids is called the lateral canthus.

The lacrimal system of the eye consists of the tear-producing meibomian glands (located on the lid margins), the lacrimal glands (located in the lateral area of the upper lids), and smaller lacrimal glands (located along the upper fornix). The lacrimal glands produce the aqueous (watery) layer of the tear film. The mucin layer of the tear film is produced by the goblet cells in the conjunctiva. The oil layer is produced by the meibomian glands of the lids.

The lacrimal system also includes the tear drainage system, which starts at the puncta (tiny openings) located nasally on the upper and lower lids. These are the entrances to the upper and lower canaliculi (drainage tubes). These canaliculi join together and drain into the lacrimal sac, which in turn drains into the nasolacrimal duct that empties into the nasal cavity.

Infections and Inflammations

Urgent

Preseptal cellulitis is characterized by swelling and infection of the lid tissue in front of the orbital septum. (The orbital septum is the fibrous membrane that supports the eyelid structure and forms a barrier between the eyelids and bony orbit. It protects the lids from orbital fat pushing forward into them, and protects the orbit from lid inflammations.) The skin and lids may be tender and red, but vision, pupils, and ocular motility are normal. In contrast, orbital cellulitis does affect vision and motility as the contents of the orbit swell, while also causing lid swelling (see Chapter 2). The most common causes of preseptal cellulitis are *Staphylococcus aureus* and streptococci organisms.

Treatment is with oral and/or intravenous antibiotics, lid ointment, and warm compresses.

While preseptal cellulitis is not an emergent situation, unless the symptoms rule out orbital cellulitis, the patient should be seen on a same day basis.

Nonemergent

An external hordeolum (or stye) is an infection in an oil gland of a lash follicle. An external hordeolum is an infection of a meibomian gland on the inner lid margin. A chalazion is an internal hordeolum that has become chronic and has a formed a solid, painless lump (Figure 2-1). All of these can cause redness and swelling of the lids. Sometimes these conditions will resolve on

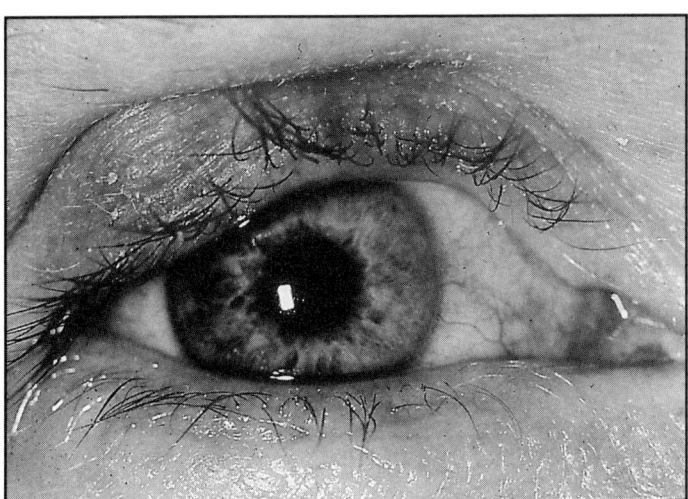

Figure 2-1. Chalazion, upper lid. (Photograph courtesy of TD Lindquist, MD, PhD.)

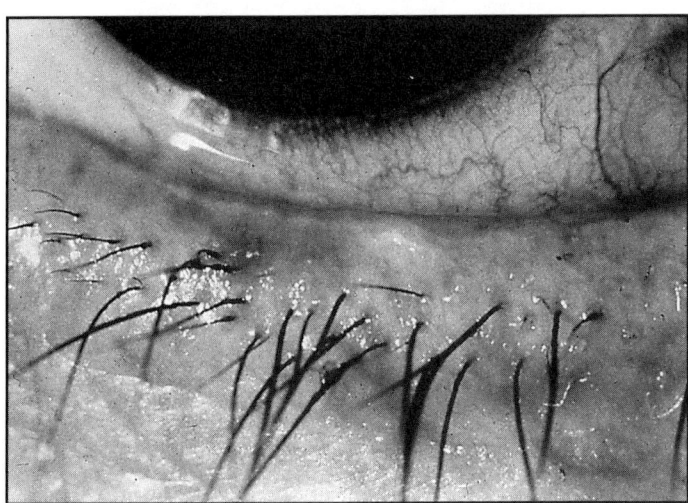

Figure 2-2. Blepharitis. (Photograph courtesy of TD Lindquist, MD, PhD.)

their own, or warm compresses and antibiotic ointments may be used as treatment to speed their resolution. In the case of chalazions, surgical curettage may be necessary.

Blepharitis is a chronic infection of the lid margin and can cause irritation, itching, and redness (Figure 2-2). Treatment involves careful daily cleaning of the eyelids, the use of warm compresses, and sometimes antibiotic ointments.

Nasolacrimal duct obstruction is a condition in which a tear duct becomes blocked, producing tearing, pain, swelling, and redness. Mucopurulent material may be expressed by pressing on the lacrimal sac. If antibiotics are ineffective, a surgical procedure to open the duct may be necessary.

These conditions are not vision-threatening, but can be uncomfortable to the patient.

Abnormalities of the Eyelids

Entropion, Ectropion, and Trichiasis

Entropion (an inward turning of the eyelid that can cause the lashes to rub the eye) (Figure 2-3), and ectropion (an outward turning of the eyelid that can cause exposure of the anterior

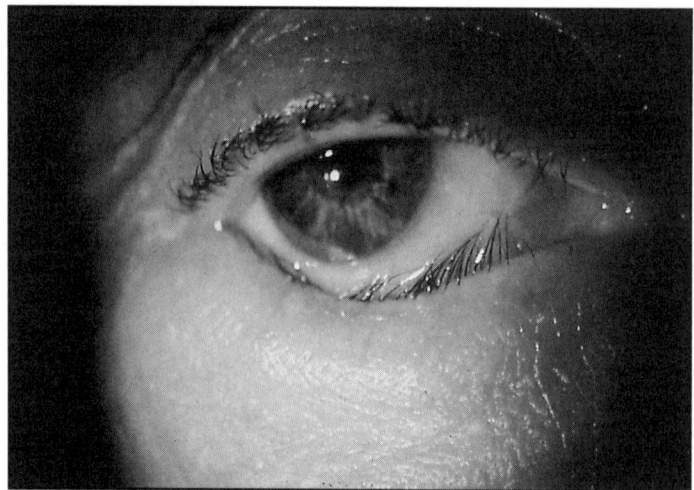

Figure 2-3. Entropion. (Photograph courtesy of EL Hargis, MD.)

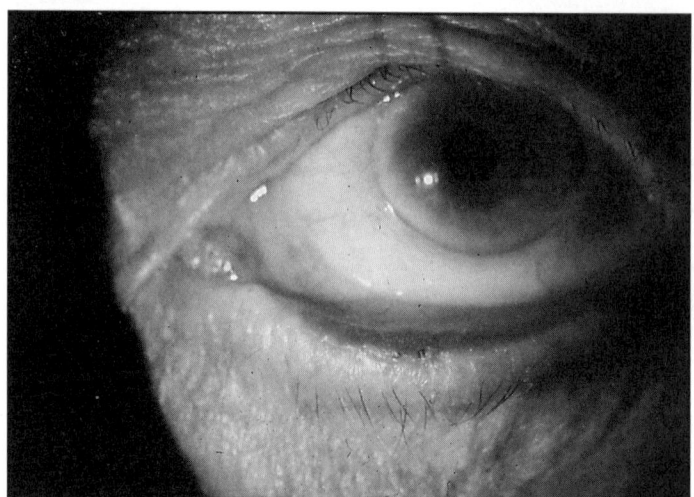

Figure 2-4. Ectropion. (Photograph courtesy of EL Hargis, MD.)

cornea and conjunctiva) (Figure 2-4) are physical abnormalities that may bring on discomfort, tearing, and redness. Treatment is usually surgical correction.

Trichiasis (in which the eyelid is in a normal position but the lashes point inward, rubbing the eye) can cause pain, redness, and corneal damage. Temporary treatment involves simple epilation (plucking) of the offending lashes. More permanent treatment may use electrolysis (a low-level electrical charge applied to the lash root), or cryosurgery (a freezing of the general area of the lash).

The discomfort caused by these conditions may necessitate a same-day appointment.

Malignant Tumors of the Eyelids

Malignancy can only be confirmed by biopsy, and these tumors are not usually painful. Evaluation of a nonpainful lid lesion can usually be done within a week or two of the patient's phone call.

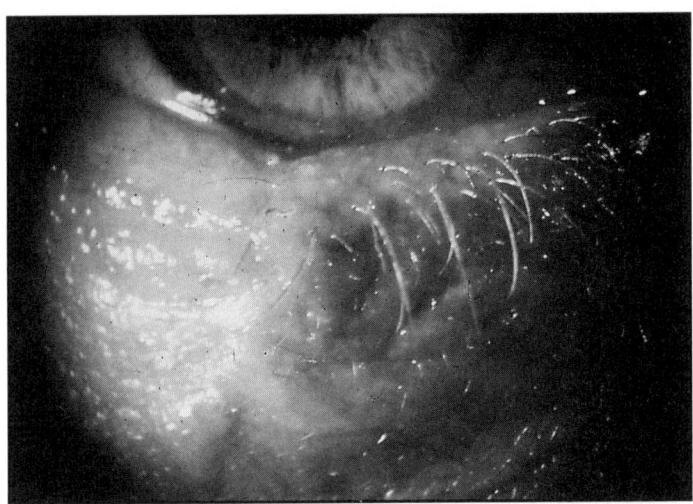

Figure 2-5. Basal cell carcinoma of lower lid. (Photograph courtesy of TD Lindquist, MD, PhD.)

Basal Cell Carcinoma

A basal cell carcinoma, or cancerous growth, is a serious condition that can develop on the lids (Figure 2-5). A malignant (health- or life-threatening) tumor may present with an inflamed, ulcerated, or dimpled surface and raised pearly edges. The patient may find the lump mildly irritating, or completely painless. While basal cell carcinomas do not metastasize (spread from their place of origin to another body area), they can be highly locally invasive. If surgical removal is performed early, a complete cure may be obtained.

Squamous Cell Carcinoma

A squamous cell carcinoma often appears similar to a basal cell carcinoma. While it can metastasize, this is uncommon. Treatment is surgical excision, and/or radiation therapy.

Sebaceous Gland Carcinoma

A sebaceous gland carcinoma usually involves the meibomian glands and can affect both upper and lower eyelids. The patient may have a history of recurrent chalazions or persistent blepharitis as the carcinoma may stimulate these conditions. Metastasis or orbital involvement can occur. Treatment is surgical excision of the carcinoma along with wide areas of tissue surrounding it.

Trauma

Blunt Trauma

Blunt trauma often causes ecchymosis of the eyelid with associated swelling and sometimes ptosis. All of these cause little, if any, lasting damage. However, any blunt ocular injury should be examined by an ophthalmologist on an urgent basis because of the risk of complications such as orbital fracture, anterior segment involvement (such as hyphema, iridodialysis, or angle recession), and retinal damage (in the form of breaks, tears and/or swelling).

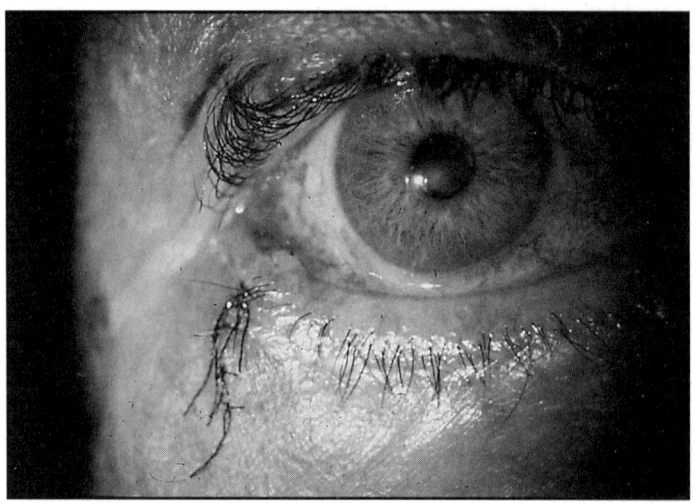

Figure 2-6. Lid laceration repair. (Photograph courtesy of EL Hargis, MD.)

Lacerations

Lacerations of the eyelids can result from automobile accidents, any high velocity projectile (such as metal or wood in carpentry work), knife wounds, animal bites, etc. Regardless of the source, a lid laceration should be seen on an emergent basis because of the risk of infection and the possibility of ocular involvement. Every patient with a lid laceration should also be examined for a globe perforation. Do not put any pressure on the eye (such as checking IOP or applying a patch) until it has been established that there is no perforation. If an ophthalmologist is not immediately available, the assistant should *lightly* patch the eye with a sterile gauze pad and notify the ophthalmologist.

Simple lid lacerations may be repaired in the office by thoroughly cleaning the wound, anesthetizing the area, removing any FBs, and suturing the wound (Figure 2-6). Anti-tetanus injection and systemic antibiotics will be prescribed.

Lid lacerations that run a high risk of contamination are sometimes cleaned and debrided of any highly infected tissue, and simply patched for a few days before suturing the wound.

Lid lacerations with ocular involvement, lacrimal drainage system involvement, or lid or ocular muscle involvement are more complicated and require surgical repair in an operating room. This is especially true if the punctum or canaliculus are involved in a laceration of the lower lid. If the openings are not repaired properly, the tears will not drain adequately. The patient will have a permanent problem with epiphora since the natural tear drainage system no longer exists.

Each layer of the lid (the skin, the muscle, the tarsus, and conjunctiva) is closed separately when suturing the lid. The sutures are usually left in place anywhere from 4 to 14 days.

Burns

A burn of any type to the eye or surrounding tissue should be seen on an emergent basis.

Chemical Burns

Chemical burns of the eyelids occur most commonly as a result of contact with solutions containing alkali (such as in ammonia, oven cleaners, and drain cleaners) or acid (such as bleach and battery fluid) that have been splashed or rubbed on the eyelid. Very often ocular involvement is also present. Initial treatment is immediate, copious rinsing of the eye and lid with water for 20 minutes before the patient leaves the scene of the splash. Rinsing should then continue with saline or water for another 20 minutes when the patient arrives at the clinic. An antibacterial ointment may be used afterward to prevent infection. (See Chapter 4 for more information on ocular involvement of chemical burns).

Thermal Burns

Most thermal burns (those involving heat or flame) are limited to the face and lids with little or no ocular involvement because of our strong blink reflex and natural instinct to protect our face with our hands.

Burns are classified as first-degree, second-degree, or third-degree, depending on the depth of the burn. A first-degree burn involves only the epidermis (the surface layer of skin) and is superficial (such as a mild sunburn). A second-degree burn is a little deeper, involving both the epidermis and a portion of the dermis (the layer of skin directly beneath the epidermis), and often results in pain and some blistering (such as occurs with a deep sunburn or scalding from hot liquids). A third-degree burn is the most severe, involving all skin layers and destroying the nerves and vascular system of the skin. Third-degree burns are often free of pain and blisters because of nerve and blood vessel destruction. Occasionally, a fourth-degree category of burns is used by some when there is also muscle involvement. Very often burns will be a combination of the different categories.

As with any lid injury, an ophthalmic exam needs to be performed as soon as possible because, as swelling of the lids increases, the difficulty of the exam also increases. If there is involvement of the meibomian glands and/or conjunctiva, corneal dryness may become a concern.

As the swelling subsides, there is a danger that a cicatricial ectropion may develop, in which the eyelid is pulled away from the eye by scar tissue, resulting in exposure keratitis. If this occurs, a tarsorrhaphy may be performed, where the upper and lower eyelids are partially or fully stitched together (usually on a temporary basis). This may help decrease the possibility that the tarsal plate will twist or distort, and also helps protect the cornea from drying.

Chapter 3

Emergencies and Injuries of the Orbit

Linda Sims, COT

KEY POINTS

- Orbital injuries often result in proptosis, restriction of ocular motility, diplopia, and/or eyelid swelling.
- Orbital blow-out fractures occur when blunt trauma fractures the thin bones of the orbit, possibly allowing the eye muscles and/or globe to be displaced into a sinus cavity.
- Intraorbital FBs may result in serious eye complications or cause no problem at all.
- Orbital cellulitis, an infection of the orbital contents, may be life- or sight-threatening.

Anatomy of the Orbit

The bony orbit of the eye (Figure 3-1) is a cone- or pear-shaped opening made up of seven bones that serve to house and protect the eye, ocular muscles, nerves, and blood vessels. The orbit also contains orbital fat, which serves to further protect and cushion the contents of the orbit. The paraorbital sinuses are located superiorly, inferiorly, and medially to the orbit. The optic and sympathetic nerves and the ophthalmic artery pass through the orbit posteriorly at the optic foramen (an opening in the sphenoid bone). Other nerves and blood vessels pass through the thin medial wall through small foramina (openings) and fissures between the orbital bones.

The roof of the orbit is formed by two bones; the lesser wing of the sphenoid bone and the frontal bone. These bones are relatively thick and therefore stronger than the bones of the orbital floor and medial area.

The floor of the orbit is made up of three bones: the zygomatic, maxillary, and palatine bones. These bones are thin and thus weak. "Blow-out fractures" occur when blunt trauma fractures these thin bones. The floor of the orbit also makes up the roof of the air-containing maxillary sinus, which offers no support to the orbit floor.

The lateral wall of the orbit (located temporally) consists of the greater wing of the sphenoid and the zygomatic bones. While this area is relatively strong, only the posterior globe is protected by it, leaving the anterior globe more vulnerable to blows from the side.

The medial wall (located nasally) is made up of four bones; the maxillary, lacrimal, ethmoid, and sphenoid bones. These bones are thin and, like the orbital floor, more vulnerable to fractures.

Orbital Blow-Out Fractures

Fractures of the bones of the orbital floor and medial orbital area occur as a result of blunt trauma, usually by an object larger than the orbit, such as a fist, golf ball, or hammer. They may also occur in motor vehicle accidents. The force of the blow pushes the eye back into the socket, increasing the pressure on the orbital bones. Because the bones of the floor and medial wall are thin, they break relatively easily. The breaking of the bones actually dissipates the force of the blow, lessening the chance that the globe will be ruptured.

If the floor of the orbit is no longer intact, the inferior oblique and inferior rectus muscles may protrude through the break and into the maxillary sinus cavity, restricting eye movement. On rare occasions, the globe itself may sink into the maxillary sinus cavity (a condition known as enophthalmus). The roof and lateral orbital areas can be involved in fractures, but this is less common.

A patient who has experienced a non-penetrating blunt trauma may have symptoms of ecchymosis, edema, exophthalmos (a bulging forward of the eyeball) secondary to edema, orbital emphysema (air from the sinuses entering the orbit), subconjunctival hemorrhage, and ptosis. If enophthalmus occurs, it usually does not develop until 7 to 10 days after the trauma, when the edema begins to subside. There may also be diplopia and restricted eye movements that can be secondary to muscle entrapment (as discussed above), muscle injury, edema, and/or hemorrhage of the orbital fat. Facial involvement may also be present in the form of numbness of the lower lid, and side of the nose, as well as the cheek, upper lip, and gums due to nerve trauma.

Consider the possibility of a blow-out fracture any time a patient with a "black eye" is seen, especially if diplopia is present. A patient phoning the office with a blunt trauma incident should be seen on an urgent basis.

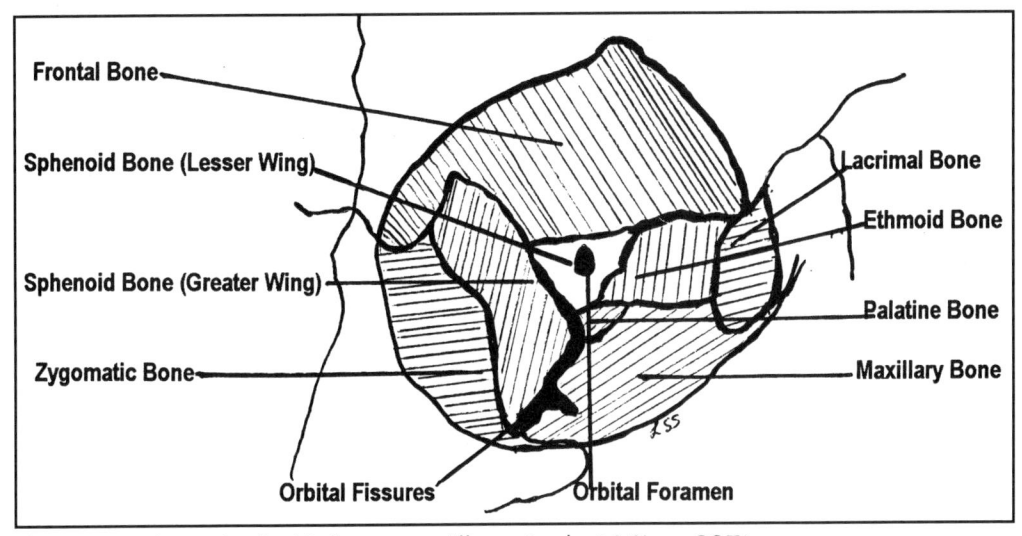

Figure 3-1. Schematic of orbital anatomy. (Illustration by LS Sims, COT.)

Once the patient arrives at the office, put no pressure on the globe until the ophthalmologist has determined that the globe has not been ruptured or perforated. Check vision and obtain a complete history of the incident (what happened, when it occurred, any treatment prior to arrival), along with the usual patient history. EOM function tests, globe displacement tests, and IOP tests will also need to be performed per your ophthalmologist's instruction.

Necessary diagnostic tests may include a CT scan of the orbits and brain. If there is restriction of eye movement and/or diplopia for more than a week, a forced duction test may be performed (in which an anesthetized muscle is grasped and the eye rotated to see if there is restriction of movement).

Treatment may include oral antibiotics and steroids, nasal decongestants, and cold packs for 1 to 2 days. The patient should be instructed not to blow his or her nose due to the chance of forcing infected sinus contents into the orbit. If diplopia persists after the swelling has subsided, if a large fracture is present, or if post-trauma cosmesis is unacceptable, surgery may be performed. The patient should also be counseled as to symptoms of RD and orbital cellulitis. If surgical repair is needed, it is not usually performed for at least 1 week after trauma, to allow for the acute orbital edema to subside.

Intraorbital Foreign Bodies

FBs that have become lodged within the orbit may never cause ocular problems, or symptoms may appear days to years later. Symptoms can include decreased vision, double vision, pain, or infection. There may or may not be swelling, eyelid ecchymosis, laceration of the lids or conjunctiva, proptosis, and limited motility. If the optic nerve has been affected, there may be an afferent pupillary defect.

The type of material that makes up the FB often determines the signs and symptoms, as well as the course of treatment. Organic material, such as plant and wood particles, are poorly tolerated by the eye. The rate of infection is also very high with such materials. The eye will also not tolerate any FB with a high copper content. (Copper alloys, however, such as brass and bronze,

Figure 3-2. Orbital cellulitis. (Photograph courtesy of Paula Parker, COMT.)

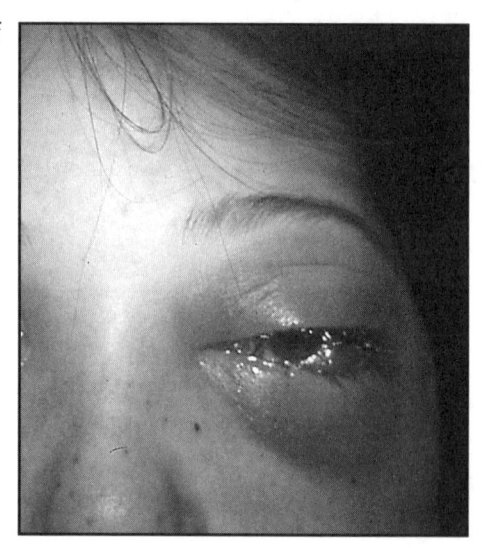

are better tolerated and may only produce slight inflammation.) Materials considered inert (or nonreactive), such as glass, plastic, stone, and most metals, are usually well tolerated and only need to be removed if they cause decreased ocular motility, diplopia, or scleral or retinal swelling.

CT scans are helpful in determining the location of an FB and whether or not the globe has been ruptured. MRI's may be used for detection of a wooden or other organic FB, but should not be used if the FB is suspected to be metal. Ultrasound B-scans may also be used to locate an FB. If there is any ocular drainage, a culture may be done to rule out infection.

Treatment may include oral antibiotics, tetanus vaccination, and surgical removal of the FB. If immediate surgery is not required, the patient may simply be monitored closely until a decision is made whether or not it is safe to leave the FB in the eye.

Orbital Cellulitis

Orbital cellulitis is an infection of the orbital tissues that most commonly travels to the orbit from an infection in the sinus area, a dental abscess, or elsewhere in the body (Figure 3-2). Infection of the orbital tissues can also follow trauma, sometimes not appearing until months afterward if an orbital FB has been retained.

Streptococci and staphylococci are the most common infecting organisms. Orbital cellulitis can be sight- and/or life-threatening due to the possibility of the infection spreading to the brain, and should be treated as an emergent condition.

Signs and symptoms include swollen, red lids and conjunctiva, proptosis, impaired ocular motility, pain with eye movement, double vision, fever, and headache. Vision may also be impaired, especially if the optic nerve is involved.

CT scans may show if the sinuses are also infected. Cultures will help to determine the type of organism involved.

Treatment includes hospitalization and intravenous antibiotics, later changing to oral antibiotics as the condition improves. Surgical drainage of any existing abscess may also be necessary. If corneal exposure results from proptosis, an ointment such as erythromycin may also be prescribed.

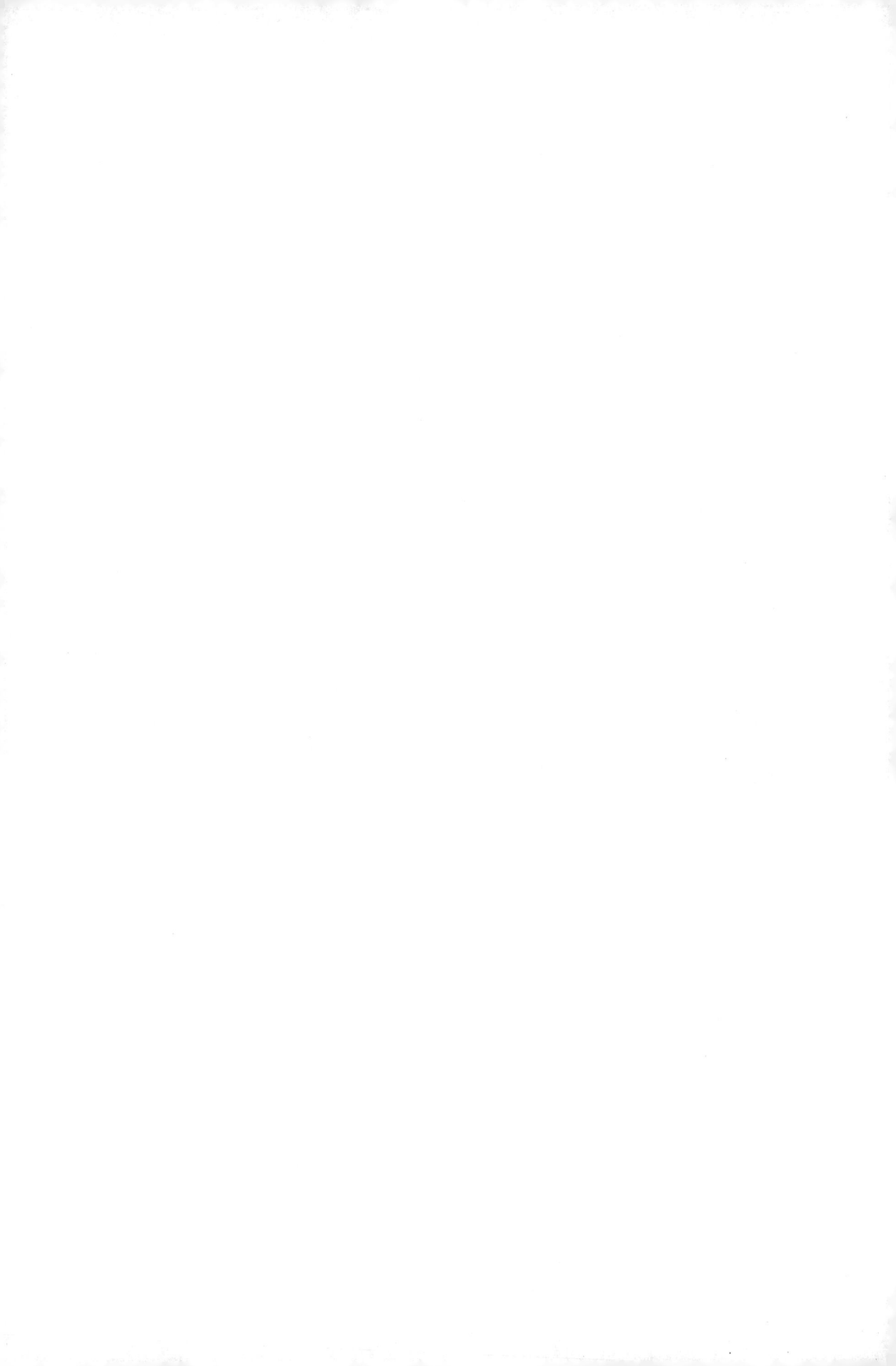

Chapter 4

Emergencies and Injuries of the Conjunctiva, Sclera, and Cornea

Linda Sims, COT

KEY POINTS

- The conjunctiva is a clear vascular tissue that supplies the eyelids and sclera with oxygen and nutrients.
- Most cases of conjunctivitis are not urgent, but there are some exceptions (such as gonococcal conjunctivitis).
- The sclera is the white, opaque, elastic collagen tissue that encompasses the globe from the cornea to the optic nerve, giving the eye its shape and form.
- Scleritis, an inflammation of the sclera, can cause extreme pain and photophobia and lead to perforation of the globe.
- The cornea is the clear avascular structure at the front of the eye that must remain clear for good vision.
- The cornea contains thousands of nerve endings and therefore is very sensitive to touch or injury.
- Corneal injuries or infections should usually be seen on an urgent basis because of the cornea's vital role in maintaining good vision.
- Chemical burns are an emergency and the patient must be instructed to flush the eye for at least 20 minutes before leaving for treatment.
- Conjunctival and corneal foreign bodies need to be seen on an urgent or emergent basis.
- Lacerations of ocular tissues are usually an emergency situation.

Conjunctiva

Anatomy

The conjunctiva is the clear mucous membrane that lines the eyelids and covers the outer sclera. The portion of conjunctiva that lines the eyelids is called the palpebral conjunctiva. The portion covering the outer sclera is known as the bulbar conjunctiva. The fornix is the junction beneath the upper and lower eyelids where the bulbar and palpebral conjunctiva meet and form a pocket of tissue. The conjunctival tissue contains a multitude of fine blood vessels that supply oxygen and nourishment to both the eyelids and scleral tissues.

Conjunctivitis

Conjunctivitis is characterized by ocular redness (conjunctival injection), grittiness, itching, burning, and discharge (which usually builds up during sleep, making the lids difficult to open in the morning) (Figure 4-1). Its causes include viral or bacterial infections, allergies, and environmental sources. The type of discharge can help to differentiate the cause. Acute conjunctivitis is usually caused by bacteria and has a mucopurulent discharge (which is thick, containing mucus and pus). In contrast, a watery discharge is characteristic of viral conjunctivitis, and a watery discharge with white, stringy mucus suggests an allergic conjunctivitis (see Chapter 9).

Most cases are diagnosed and treated by clinical signs and symptoms alone. While conjunctivitis may cause the patient some discomfort, usually the symptoms will come and go without medical treatment. Most cases are neither emergent or urgent. However, there are exceptions.

Gonococcal Conjunctivitis

Gonococcal conjunctivitis is a severe ocular infection that can lead to corneal ulceration, perforation, and blindness if treatment is delayed (Figure 4-2). The patient with suggestive signs and symptoms should be seen on an urgent basis. The infection is characterized by a large amount of purulent discharge, chemosis (conjunctival swelling), and papillae (small elevations on the palpebral conjunctiva). It is caused by the same bacterial organism that causes gonorrhea, so the patient and his or her sexual contacts need to be evaluated for the venereal disease. Smears and cultures may be taken to determine the type of infection. Treatment may include hospitalization, systemic and topical antibiotics, and saline rinses periodically throughout the day.

This infection can also occur in newborns who contract it during passage through the birth canal. Most countries now routinely prophylactically treat newborns with silver nitrate or antibacterial drops to prevent eye infections from the gonococci organism, as well as other organisms that can be transmitted during birth.

Viral Conjunctivitis

Viral conjunctivitis is a contagious form of conjunctivitis that can be passed from one person to another by shaking hands, sharing towels, etc. Symptoms generally start with an upper respiratory tract infection or contact with an infected person, and include a watery discharge (that may contain some mucus), swollen eyelids, eye and lid redness, and eye irritation. Symptoms tend to become more severe in the first 4 to 7 days, and may last from 2 to 3 weeks. Treatment includes the use of artificial tears, cool compresses, and vasoconstrictors or antihistamines if itching is severe. While not vision-threatening, the patient should be seen on a semi-urgent basis because of the possibility of infecting others.

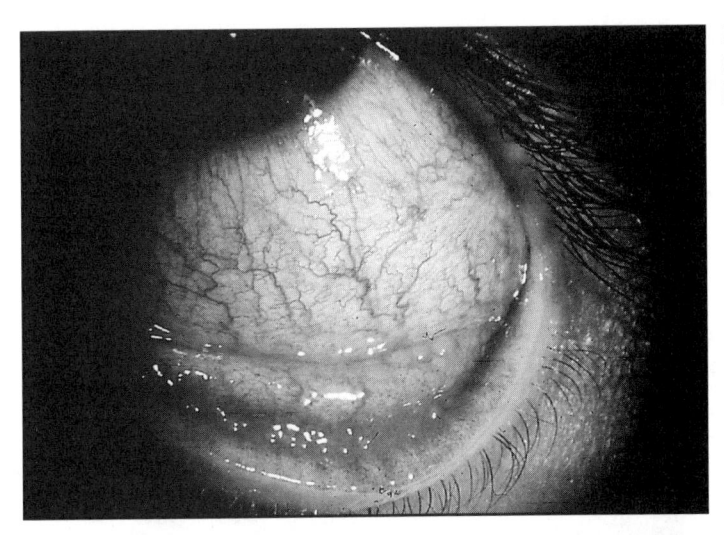

Figure 4-1. Conjunctivitis. (Photograph courtesy of TD Lindquist, MD, PhD.)

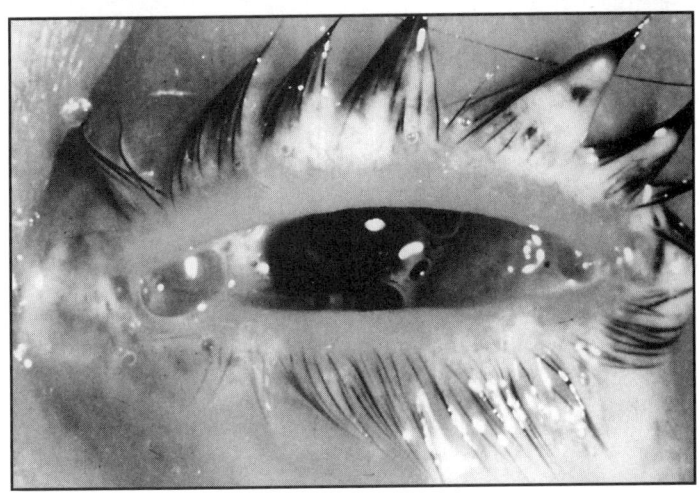

Figure 4-2. Mucopurulent conjunctivitis. (Photograph courtesy of TD Lindquist, MD, PhD.)

Sclera and Episclera

Anatomy

The sclera, or "white of the eye," is the eye's protective opaque covering that encompasses the globe from the limbus (the junction of the cornea and the sclera) to the optic nerve. The sclera consists of collagen and elastic tissue. It is able to expand or contract with variations in IOP, while still providing enough support to prevent distortion of ocular contents.

The episclera is the highly elastic, vascular, surface layer of the sclera that lies beneath the conjunctiva and attaches to Tenon's capsule (a thin membrane that attaches at the limbus and encircles the globe back to the optic nerve, and also encases the EOM tendons).

Scleritis

Scleritis is an inflammation of the sclera that can lead to scleral thinning, perforations, loss of vision, or loss of the eye (Figure 4-3). Early diagnosis and treatment are essential, so the

Figure 4-3. Scleritis. (Photograph courtesy of TD Lindquist, MD, PhD.)

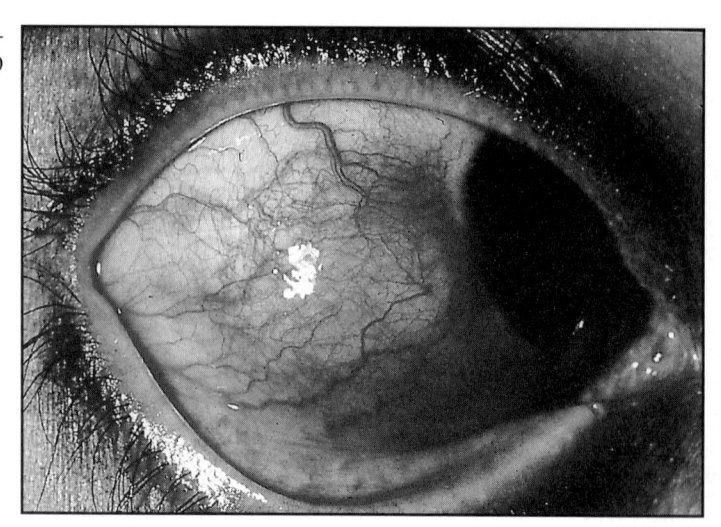

patient should be seen on an urgent basis. Symptoms usually have a gradual onset and include severe, deep pain that sometimes extends into the forehead, brow, or jaw area, and may be so intense as to awaken the patient from sleep. There may also be ocular redness, light sensitivity, tearing, and decreased vision. The sclera may appear thin and bluish, especially when viewed in natural light. The blood vessels of the sclera, episclera, and/or conjunctiva appear inflamed.

Scleritis may be differentiated from episcleritis (discussed next) by placing a drop of phenylephrine in the eye. Episcleral vessels will blanche (whiten) 10 to 15 minutes after drop instillation, indicating episcleritis. Scleral vessels will not whiten, so if the redness is still present after 10 to 15 minutes, the deeper scleral vessels are involved (indicating scleritis).

Scleritis may be accompanied by other ocular problems such as keratitis, uveitis, glaucoma, and cataracts. If the inflammation is in the posterior area of the sclera, it may not be possible for the ophthalmologist to view it directly, making diagnosis more difficult. Posterior scleritis may additionally cause proptosis, a rapid onset of hyperopia, and RDs.

Approximately half of the patients with scleritis also have connective tissue diseases (such as rheumatoid arthritis or systemic lupus) or a history of herpes zoster ophthalmicus, syphilis, or gout. Other systemic diseases less commonly associated with scleritis include tuberculosis, sarcoidosis, Lyme disease, and hypertension. The sooner these underlying causes are diagnosed, the sooner medical management can begin.

Treatment includes nonsteroidal anti-inflammatory drugs (NSAIDs, such as ibuprofen), systemic steroids, and sometimes topical steroids (for patient comfort). Surgery is rarely needed. In some cases, the patient may be referred to a rheumatologist for systemic treatment and consideration of immunosuppression therapy. If there is significant scleral thinning, the patient should wear eyeglasses or a protective shield to lessen the risk of perforation due to trauma.

Episcleritis

Episcleritis is an inflammation of the episcleral layer (Figure 4-4). Symptoms include a sudden onset of redness, photophobia, mild pain in one or both eyes. The problem tends to recur. If it becomes chronic, purple nodules with surrounding swelling may develop. Usually, episcleritis

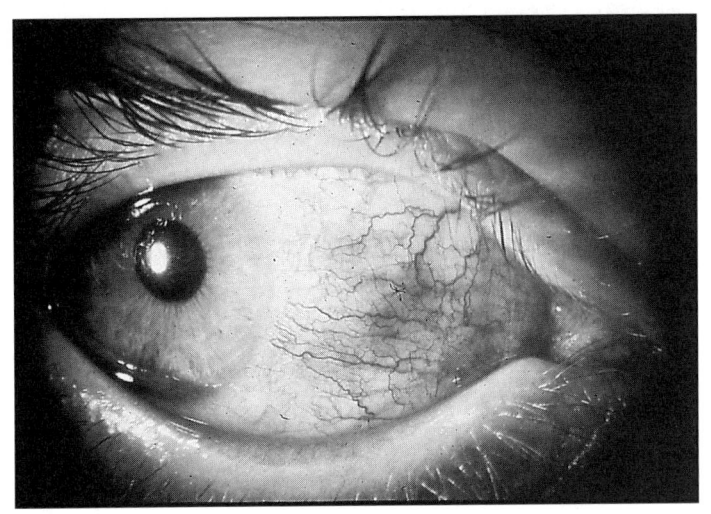

Figure 4-4. Episcleritis. (Photograph courtesy of TD Lindquist, MD, PhD.)

is transient with no lasting effect, but because the episcleral layer is also affected when scleritis is present, the patient should be seen on an urgent basis.

Treatment includes artificial tears or a topical vasoconstrictor for mild cases, topical steroids for moderate or severe cases, and occasionally NSAIDs.

Cornea

Anatomy

The cornea is the transparent, avascular structure at the front of the eye that provides approximately two-thirds of the eye's refractive ability (the lens provides the other third). It also serves to protect the inner eye from bacteria, dirt, and other foreign material.

The cornea is thinnest at its center (about 0.5 mm) and thickest at its edges (approximately 1 mm). It can be divided into five separate layers (from outside to inside): the epithelium, Bowman's layer, the stroma, Descemet's membrane, and the endothelium (Figure 4-5).

The epithelium is the surface corneal layer. It is made up of approximately five layers of cells and thousands of nerve endings. These nerve endings are responsible for the sensation of pain when the cornea is touched or injured. The epithelium's main functions are to protect the eye and other corneal layers from foreign material and to absorb oxygen and nutrients from the tears.

Bowman's layer anchors the epithelium to the stroma and does not regenerate when injured. Any injury that descends to Bowman's layer or beyond will scar when healed.

The stroma is the main body of the cornea, making up approximately 90% of its thickness. It is comprised of water, protein fibers, and cells. The stroma gives the cornea its strength, shape, and elasticity.

Descemet's membrane lies between the stroma and the endothelium and is made up of a fine mesh of collagen fibers that provides rigidity to the cornea.

The endothelium is the posterior layer of the cornea. It is made up of a single layer of cells that pump the excess water from the stroma, helping to maintain the cornea's clarity. Endothelial cells are lost both as we age and from some corneal conditions (such as Fuch's dystrophy).

Figure 4-5. Schematic of corneal anatomy. (Illustration by LS Sims, COT.)

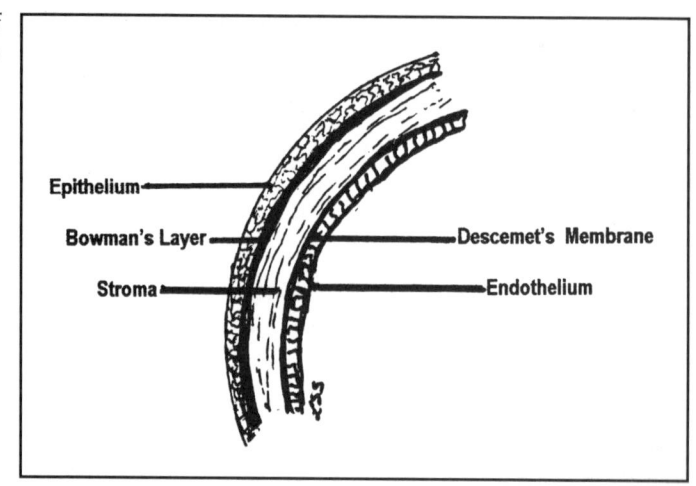

Because these cells do not regenerate, remaining cells expand to fill in space left by lost cells. If enough cells are lost, the endothelium's pumping function is diminished. This can lead to corneal edema and decompensation, which may lead to the need for a corneal transplant.

When endothelial cell loss is suspected, specular microscopy may be performed in which the endothelial cells are photographed. This provides an estimated cell count, as well as the size, shape, and distribution of endothelial cells (Figure 4-6).

Pachymetry measurements, by means of ultrasound or optical instruments, provide corneal thickness readings. These readings can suggest an endothelial defect (normal central corneal thickness usually ranges from approximately 0.50 to 0.55 mm, while endothelial disease may be indicated when the reading is in the 0.60 mm range).

Injuries, abrasions, and ulcers cause pain, tearing, redness, photophobia, and blurred vision. The deeper the involvement penetrates, the greater the severity of symptoms. Corneal opacification and decreased acuity can result when the deeper layers are affected. Because of the cornea's important role in good vision, and because of the pain and discomfort associated with corneal injury, the patient with the following corneal disorders should be seen on at least an urgent basis.

Urgent Conditions

Recurrent Corneal Erosion

Recurrent corneal erosion occurs when healing epithelium fails to adhere to Bowman's layer (Figure 4-7). This may happen after an abrasion (a scratch or scrape) has healed, and may be associated with previous chemical injury, previous eye surgery, infections, or dry eye.

The patient may experience an FB sensation or ocular pain when waking. This is due to a re-abrading of the epithelial layer when opening the lids or rubbing the eye. Other symptoms include ocular redness, photophobia, and tearing. Treatment may include cycloplegic drops for comfort, as well as an antibiotic ointment. In acute cases, a pressure patch may be used for 24 to 48 hours. After the epithelium is healed, artificial tear ointments and drops are prescribed. In cases where the epithelium is loose and not healing, debridement (removal of the affected tissue to aid healing) may be done. In some instances, the excimer laser is being used to ablate the affected tissue. If the erosion is unresponsive to other treatments, a bandage soft contact lens may be prescribed for several months.

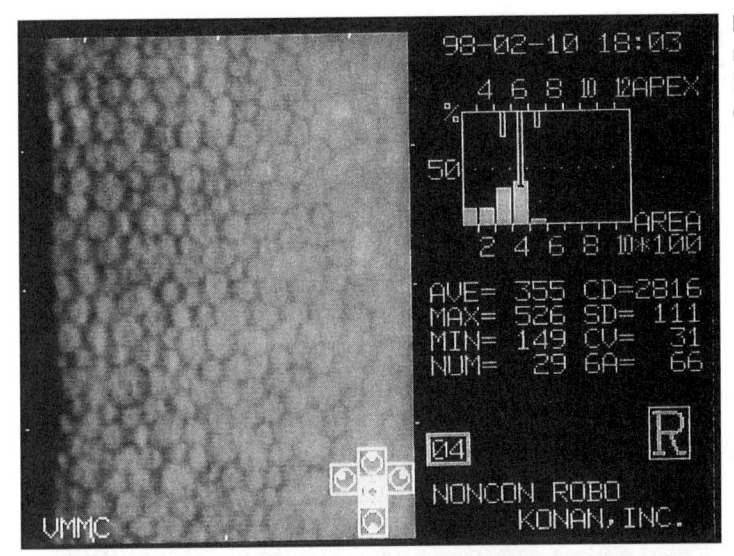

Figure 4-6. Specular microscopy, showing endothelial cells in a healthy cornea. (Courtesy of LS Sims, COT.)

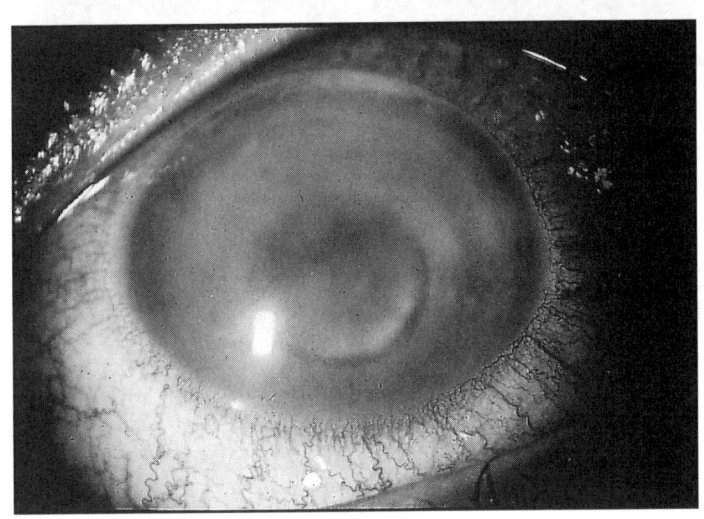

Figure 4-7. Recurrent erosion. (Photograph courtesy of TD Lindquist, MD, PhD.)

Keratitis

Keratitis is a corneal inflammation in which the cornea loses some transparency and its cells become infiltrated, sometimes resulting in corneal ulcers (Figure 4-8). Its causes include viral or bacterial organisms, chemical or physical injury, or high levels of ultraviolet light exposure.

Corneal ulcers occur when the area of corneal tissue loss penetrates the epithelial layer and extends into the stroma (Figure 4-9). Corneal infiltrates are white opacities in the stromal layer and occur when there is an abnormal accumulation of fluid and cells. Ulcers and infiltrates can be caused by viral, bacterial, or fungal organisms, or trauma.

Infectious Corneal Keratitis/Ulcers

Ocular Herpes

Ocular herpes is caused by an infection of the herpes simplex virus (usually HSV I, the same virus responsible for cold sores). It is characterized by branch-shaped corneal erosions (dendrites)

Figure 4-8. Keratitis. (Photograph courtesy of TD Lindquist, MD, PhD.)

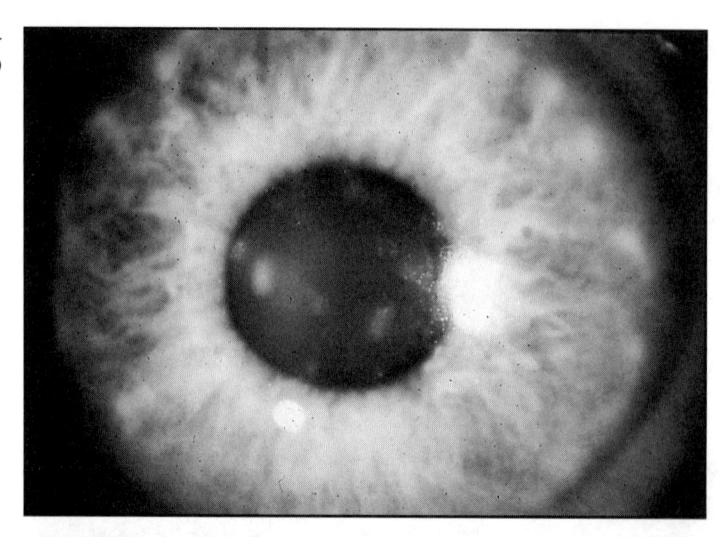

Figure 4-9. Corneal ulcer with distortion of the slit beam. (Photograph courtesy of EL Hargis, MD.)

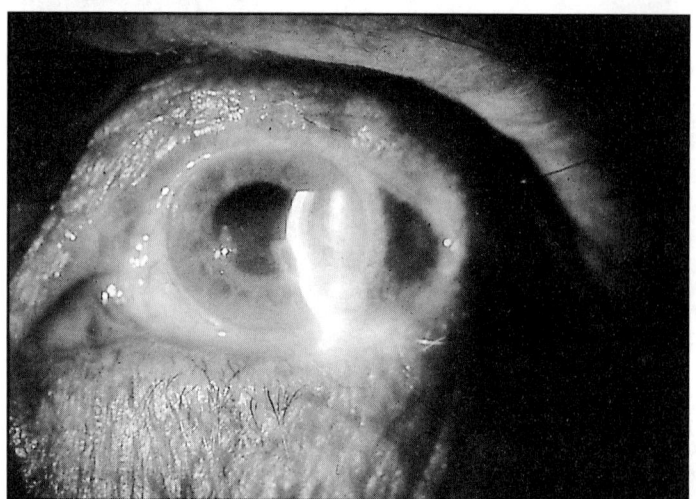

that can develop into corneal ulcers that penetrate into the stroma and may result in scarring and/or intraocular infection (Figure 4-10). The virus remains dormant the majority of the time, but may reactivate secondary to such things as stress, trauma, steroid use, or sunlight exposure. Symptoms are often unilateral and include pain, an FB sensation, redness, tearing, blurred vision, and photophobia. There may also be a rash on the eyelids as well as conjunctivitis or uveitis. Recurrent episodes can result in a significant vision decrease over the years. Smears and cultures may be done to confirm the diagnosis. Treatment includes anti-viral medications and sometimes debridement of the affected tissue.

Herpes Zoster Virus

Herpes zoster virus (HZV) is the virus that causes chicken pox. After the initial "chicken pox" infection, the virus becomes dormant. When the virus is re-activated (usually during adulthood) it travels down nerve fibers of some areas of the body. It may travel to the head and neck, where it can involve the eye, nose, mouth, cheek, and forehead. This reactivated disorder is known as shingles. Shingles involves a blistering skin rash, fever, and painful inflammation of the nerve fiber. (The pain continues even after the rash has cleared.)

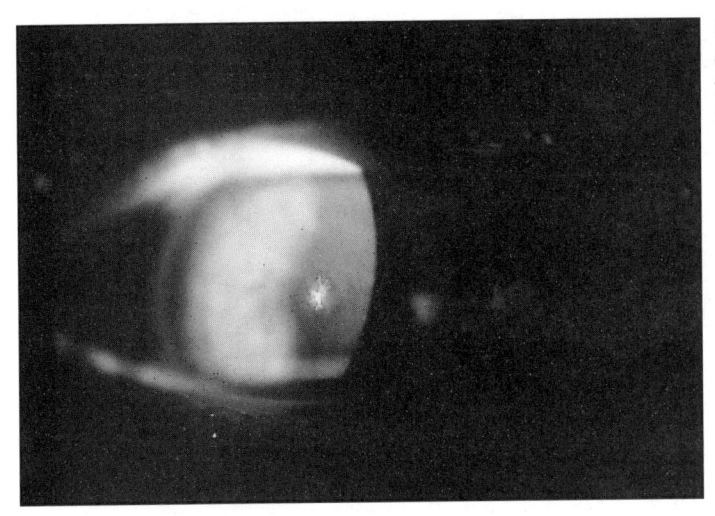

Figure 4-10. Herpetic corneal dendrite. (Photograph courtesy of TD Lindquist, MD, PhD.)

When the eye becomes involved, symptoms include redness, blurred vision, and ocular pain. About 40% of those infected with shingles in the facial area will have corneal involvement. This includes corneal inflammation and lesions, which, if left untreated, can invade the stroma and cause scarring (Figure 4-11). Ocular involvement may also result in conjunctival involvement, uveitis, scleritis, secondary glaucoma, retinitis, optic neuritis, and cranial nerve palsy. Standard treatment includes anti-viral medications. Other specific ocular findings (such as secondary glaucoma) may also be treated.

HZV can be spread through inhalation and is contagious if one has not had chicken pox. Pregnant women should avoid contact with those who have chicken pox or HZV.

Bacterial Corneal Infiltrates/Ulcers

Bacteria are the most common cause of corneal infiltrates and ulcers. (Corneal infections are generally assumed to be bacterial unless there is a reason to suspect another source. Cultures can be done to aid the diagnosis.) The most common bacterial source is the *Staphylococcus aureus* organism (Figure 4-12). Symptoms include ocular redness, pain, vision decrease, light sensitivity, and discharge. This infection is treated with topical cycloplegics and antibiotics.

Fungal Keratitis

Fungal infection usually follows ocular trauma from vegetable matter (such as a plant or tree branch), but may also occur in someone with a chronic eye disease. Symptoms include pain or an FB sensation, light sensitivity, ocular redness, tearing, and mucopurulent discharge. The infiltrate may appear as a grayish-white stromal opacity with a feathery border, with or without an ulceration (Figure 4-13). There may also be smaller lesions surrounding the infiltrate. If cultures show the infection to be fungal, treatment includes cycloplegic and antifungal topical and systemic medications. Hospitalization may be considered. A fungal infection can perforate the cornea, requiring a corneal transplant. Because some ocular fungal infections can actually be life-threatening and/or sight-threatening, patients with a penetrating injury involving organic material should be seen on an emergent basis.

Acanthamoeba

Acanthamoeba is a protozoan (single-celled microorganism) that may be found in soil, fresh and salt water, swimming pools, hot tubs, and homemade contact lens solutions. Soft contact lens

Figure 4-11. Herpetic lesion. (Photograph courtesy of EL Hargis, MD.)

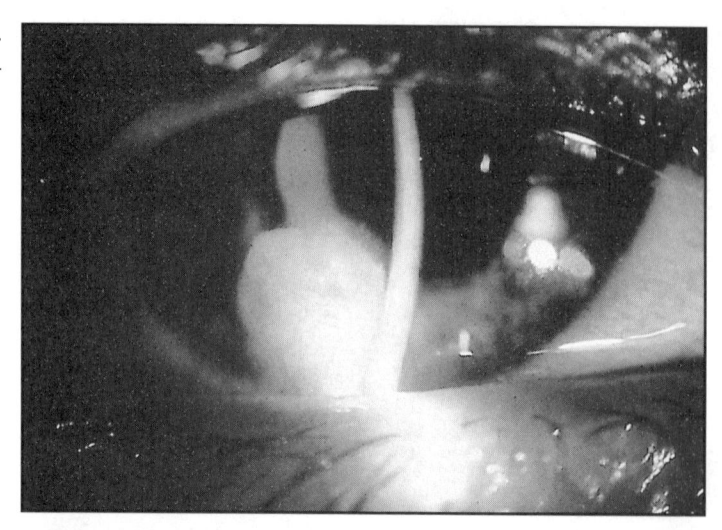

Figure 4-12. Corneal ulcer secondary to the *Staphylococcus aureus* organism. (Photograph courtesy of TD Lindquist, MD, PhD.)

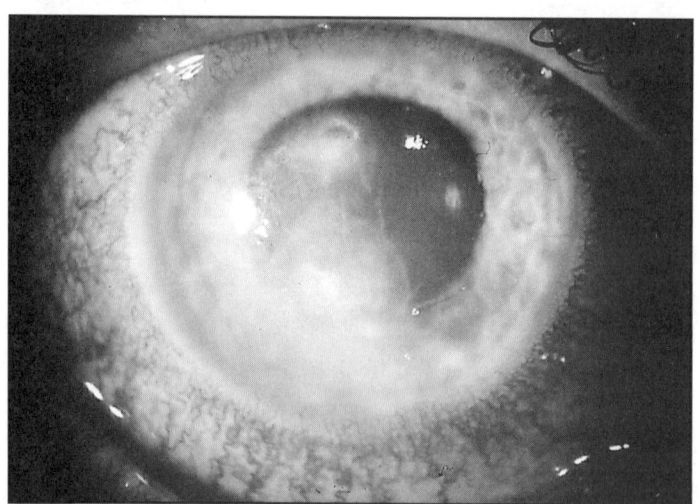

Figure 4-13. Fungal corneal ulcer. (Photograph courtesy of Paula Parker, COMT.)

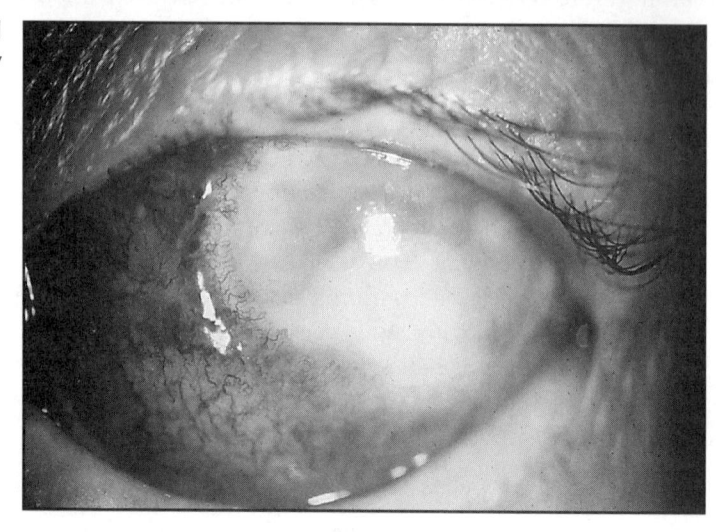

wearers are at higher risk of contracting this protozoan, especially if they swim, use a hot tub, or use non-sterile saline solutions with their contacts. Symptoms include severe ocular pain, redness, and light sensitivity. There may be eyelid swelling, as well as cells and flare in the anterior chamber. Later signs may include a ring-shaped stromal infiltrate and/or a corneal ulcer (Figure 4-14). Corneal cultures and biopsies may be performed to confirm the diagnosis. Treatment is difficult and often ineffective, but includes discontinuing contact lens wear, topical cycloplegics and antimicrobials, systemic pain medicines, and sometimes hospitalization. Despite treatment, corneal perforations sometimes result, requiring a corneal transplant; however, the protozoan may remain active in the eye and also invade the corneal graft.

Keratitis/Corneal Ulcers from Other Sources

Contact Lens Related Keratitis/Ulcers

Any contact lens wearer reporting pain, an FB sensation, and/or decreased vision (with or without ocular redness, itching, or discharge) should be seen on an urgent basis.

The most worrisome problems a contact lens wearer may encounter are corneal abrasions from poor fitting or damaged lenses and infections (bacterial, fungal, or protozoan) that may lead to corneal infiltrates and ulcers. Other sources of irritation or pain may be allergies to solution preservatives, protein deposits, insufficient oxygen reaching the cornea, corneal neovascularization, or epithelial changes (which may be due to a toxic or traumatic reaction to the contact lenses).

Treatment depends on the cause. Infections are treated as detailed above, in addition to discontinuing contact lens wear until the infection has cleared. Treatments for other problems include discontinuing contact lens wear for a time, using preservative-free artificial tears, using preservative-free contact lens solutions, and replacing or refitting the contact lenses. If the problem is due to giant papillary conjunctivitis, in which the giant papillae on the upper palpebral conjunctiva become inflamed and enlarged, contact lens wear may have to be discontinued or wearing time reduced. For more details on contact lens wear and associated problems, consult the Basic Bookshelf title *Contact Lenses*.

Corneal Graft Rejection

Corneal transplant surgery may be performed secondary to corneal degeneration, injury, or infection that has led to corneal clouding. A donor cornea is used to replace the patient's damaged cornea. Since the cornea is avascular (without blood vessels), the chances of the patient's system rejecting the foreign tissue is low. However, rejection can happen at any time, from weeks to years after surgery (Figures 4-15 and 4-16). Symptoms are a red eye, sensitivity to light, decreased vision, and/or pain. The patient should be seen on an urgent basis. With early treatment of topical (and sometimes systemic) steroids and cycloplegics, the graft may often be saved.

External Globe Trauma

Any incidence of trauma to the eye and/or surrounding tissues should be seen on an emergent basis. Each case of trauma is unique, some being very painful with obvious damage, while others are asymptomatic but still producing damage. Still others may be painful, but superficial. It is better to err on the side of caution and have the patient examined emergently.

Figure 4-14. Acanthamoeba infection showing a ring-shaped stromal infiltrate. (Photograph courtesy of TD Lindquist, MD, PhD.)

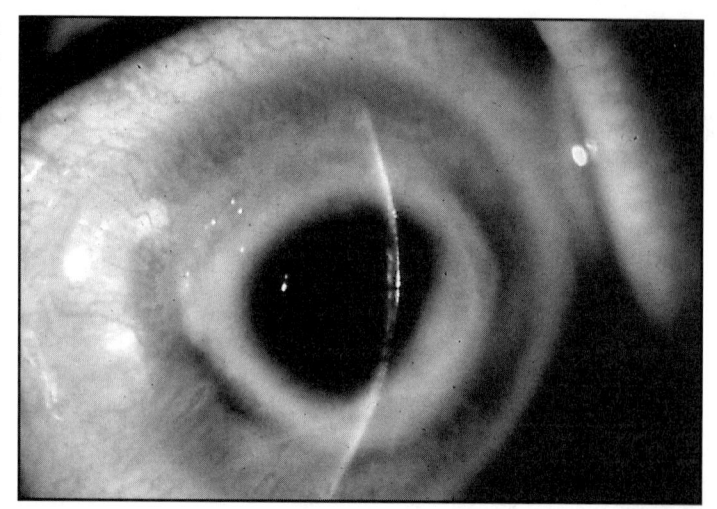

Figure 4-15. Epithelial graft rejection line. (Photograph courtesy of TD Lindquist, MD, PhD.)

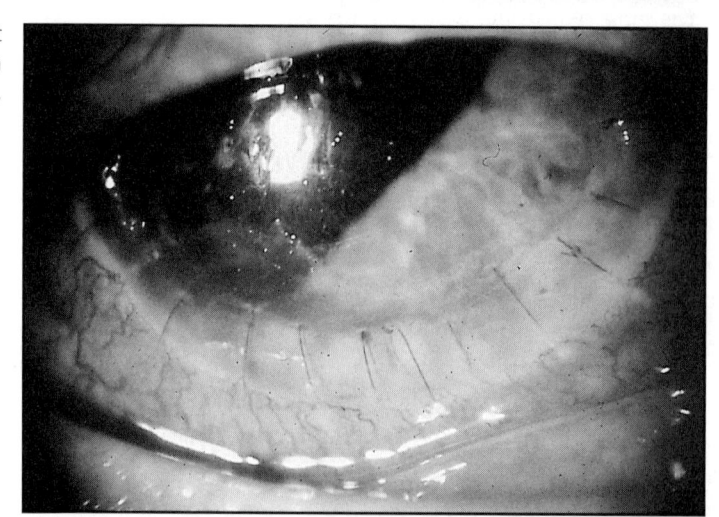

Figure 4-16. Corneal graft rejection. (Photograph courtesy of TD Lindquist, MD, PhD.)

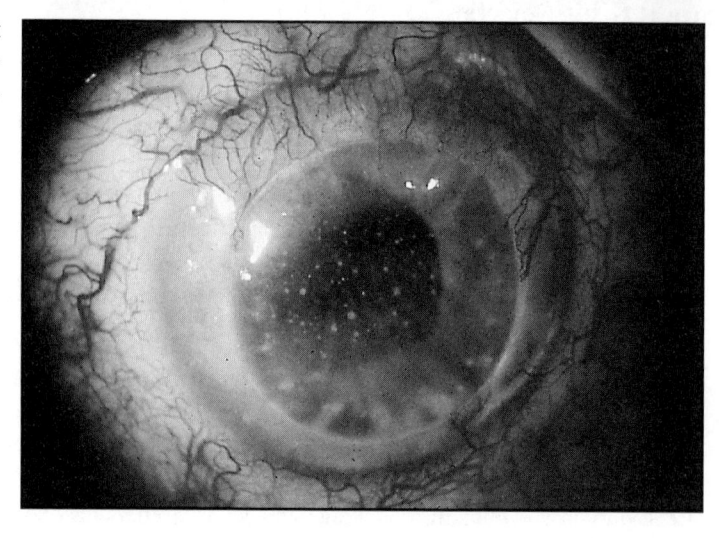

Burns

Chemical Burns

A chemical burn of the cornea and surrounding tissues is an emergency situation. Before anything else is done, the patient needs to immediately irrigate the eye and continue with irrigation for at least 20 minutes before seeking medical attention. Once arriving at the clinic or emergency room, irrigation must be continued at least another 30 minutes. Topical anesthetics, a lid speculum, and an irrigating solution connected to IV tubing may help facilitate irrigation. If the type of chemical involved is unknown, a pH paper may be helpful in determining alkalinity or acidity. The pH level of the eye should be checked 5 minutes after irrigation is stopped. If the pH level is not neutral, irrigation should be continued. After thorough irrigation, the patient's vision should be checked and details of the chemical splash obtained (what was the chemical, what time did the splash occur, what treatment occurred before the patient arrived, when did that treatment begin, etc).

Chemical burns may occur when acid- or alkali-based products or organic solvents come into contact with the eye.

Such products as ammonia, drain and oven cleaners, and calcium hydroxide (or lime, which is found in mortars, cements, and plasters) are alkaline. Alkalis are more destructive to ocular tissue than acid because the chemical reaction causes it to adhere to corneal and conjunctival tissues. Therefore, it produces immediate damage on contact and continuing damage because of the adherence.

Acid burns tend to be less destructive to ocular tissue as the acid does not form a bond with the tissues. However, acid still causes damage to the eye and immediate, copious rinsing is still required at the site of the occurrence and at the office or emergency room. Acidic products include car batteries and laboratory test chemicals. Ocular contact with these can be complicated by FBs if the incident involved an explosion.

Organic (or carbon-based) solvents include gasoline, kerosene, alcohol, and cleaning fluids, which also cause ocular damage and require the same emergency treatment as described above.

Mild to moderate chemical burns may exhibit signs ranging form slight epithelial defects to areas of complete epithelial loss, conjunctival chemosis and/or hemorrhage, anterior chamber reaction, and burns of the eyelid and periocular skin (Figure 4-17).

Moderate to severe burns show signs ranging from corneal edema to opaque corneal tissues, severe chemosis, and a greater anterior chamber reaction (Figure 4-18). However, in this case the view of the anterior chamber, iris, and lens may be occluded by an opaque cornea. There may be an increase of IOP as well as second- to third-degree burns of the eyelids and periocular skin.

Treatment includes a thorough search of the eye for FBs, debridement of necrotic tissue, a non-vasoconstrictive cycloplegic, topical antibiotics, pressure patch, and systemic pain medication. Topical steroids may be used for a short period. If IOP is elevated, systemic anti-glaucoma medications may be prescribed. If the bulbar and palpebral conjunctival tissues adhere to one another, a loosening of the tissues may be done by sweeping the fornices with a glass rod and antibiotic ointment. Hospitalization may be necessary. Cyanoacrylate adhesive may be applied to seal small perforations. A bandage soft contact lens, collagen shield, or a tarsorrhaphy may be used to help protect the cornea during healing. If the cornea continues to melt or a perforation develops, a corneal graft may be necessary.

Figure 4-17. Conjunctival chemical burn. (Photograph courtesy of EL Hargis, MD.)

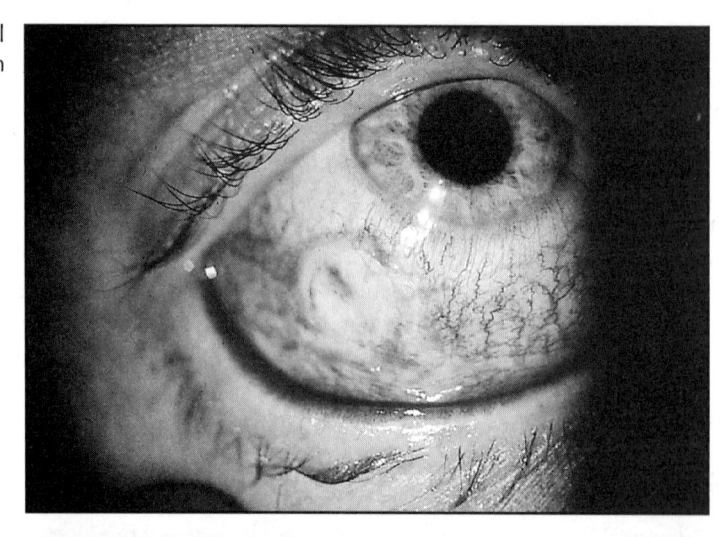

Figure 4-18. Corneal chemical burn. (Photograph courtesy of EL Hargis, MD.)

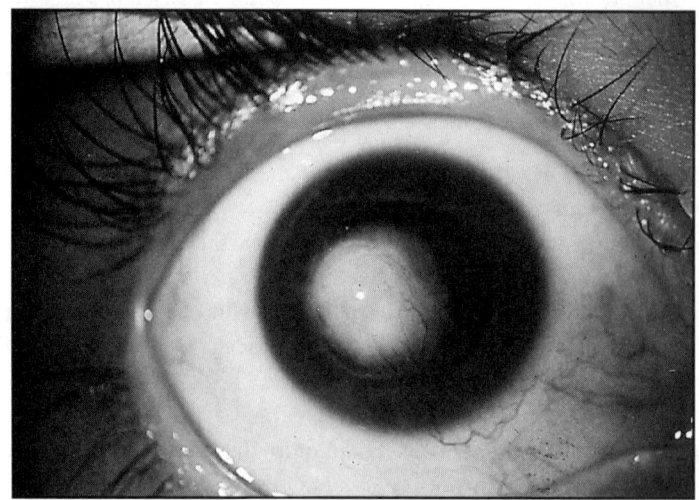

Thermal Burns

Because of our rapid blink reflex, thermal burns (caused by heat) most commonly involve the eyelids and periocular skin (see Chapter 2) rather than ocular tissue. Exceptions do occur however, from such incidences as a sudden spark or flash of flame that reaches the cornea before blinking can protect the eye (Figure 4-19). Usually the exposure is of short duration and results in superficial corneal damage that is treated with pain and topical medications.

Radiation Burns

Injuries from ultraviolet radiation usually result from exposure to sunshine, sunlamps, or welding arcs. Such a burn causes corneal damage in the form of pinpoint epithelial defects known as superficial punctate keratitis (SPK). There may be conjunctival injection, and sometimes lid and corneal edema. The patient may report using a sunlamp or welding without use of protective eyewear. Symptoms usually start 6 to 10 hours after the incident and range from an FB sensation to mild or severe pain, ocular redness, photophobia, and decreased vision. Treatment includes a topical cycloplegic, an antibiotic ointment, systemic pain medication, and a

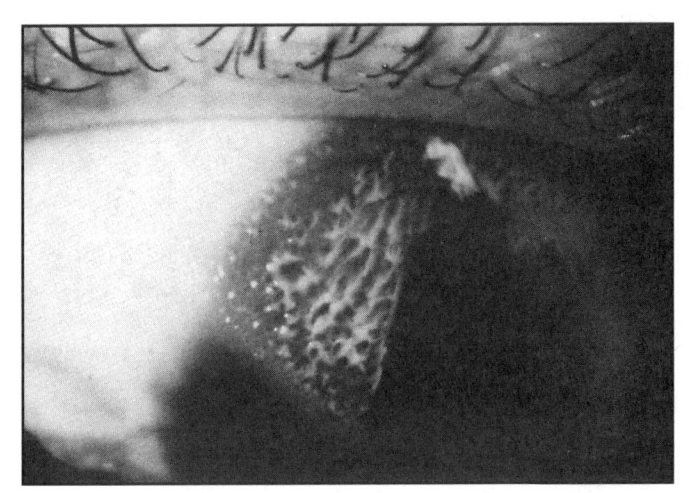

Figure 4-19. Corneal thermal burn. (Printed with permission from Herrin M. *Ophthalmic Examination and Basic Skills.* Thorofare, NJ: SLACK Incorporated; 1990.)

pressure patch for 24 hours. If the eye feels better after 24 hours, the patch is removed and the topical medications are continued. If the eye has not appreciably improved after 24 hours, the topical medications are again instilled and the eye is re-covered with a pressure patch.

Corneal Abrasion

Corneal abrasions occur when the epithelial layer is scratched or scraped by such things as a fingernail, paper, contact lens, etc, or from corneal defects caused by dry eye (Figure 4-20). Symptoms include pain or an FB sensation, redness, tearing, and blurred vision. Treatment may include topical antibiotics to prevent infection, cycloplegics for comfort, and pressure patching to allow the epithelium to heal. Abrasions usually heal quickly, within 24 to 48 hours.

Conjunctival and Corneal Foreign Bodies

Small ocular FBs are usually blinked away or washed out by tearing. Other FBs may become lodged on the cornea and bulbar or palpebral conjunctiva, requiring manual removal (Figures 4-21, 4-22, and 4-23). The patient may report symptoms of pain or an FB sensation, with tearing and/or ocular redness.

Often the patient will be able to identify an incident, such as grinding or hammering, that may have caused fragments to be projected. Be very cautious not to put any pressure on the globe especially if a projectile FB is suspected, as the projectile may have perforated the globe.

The FB may be visible either on or embedded in the cornea, or on, embedded in, or beneath the conjunctiva (if beneath the conjunctival tissue, a laceration is present). A subconjunctival hemorrhage may be evident. If the FB is metal, a rust ring may encircle it. Straight, vertical corneal scratches indicate there may be an FB under the upper eyelid that is rubbing the cornea with each blink.

During the exam, the physician will evert the eyelids to determine if there is an FB stuck to the lid. The eye will be searched for signs of perforations. Fluorescein dye from a moistened strip is placed directly over a suspected perforation site to detect leaking aqueous. If the aqueous is leaking, the fluorescein in that area will be diluted, and will appear as a green stream. This is known as Seidel's test. IOP will be checked when it is determined safe to do so. If there is an FB under the conjunctiva or a significant amount of trauma has occurred, a retinal exam will be done.

Figure 4-20. Corneal abrasion. (Photograph courtesy of TD Lindquist, MD, PhD.)

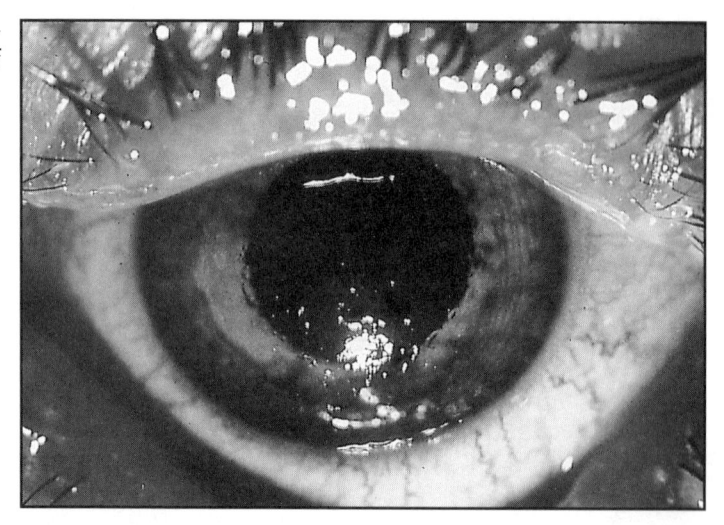

Figure 4-21. Conjunctival FB. (Photograph courtesy of TD Lindquist, MD, PhD.)

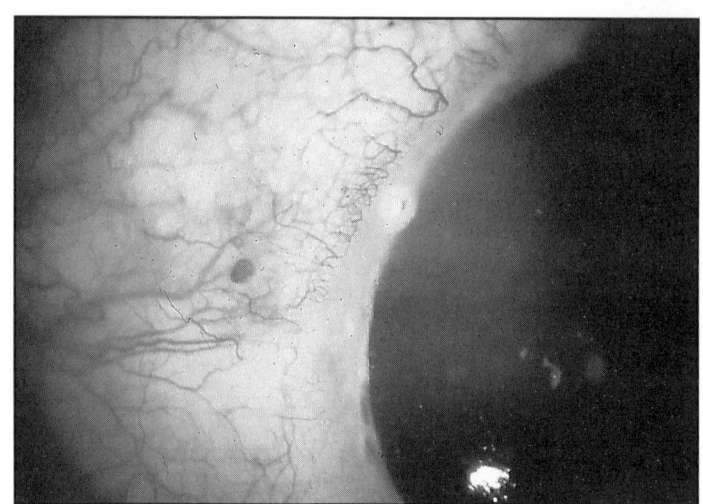

Figure 4-22. Conjunctival bug wing FB. (Photograph courtesy of Leslie Hargis-Greenshields, COMT.)

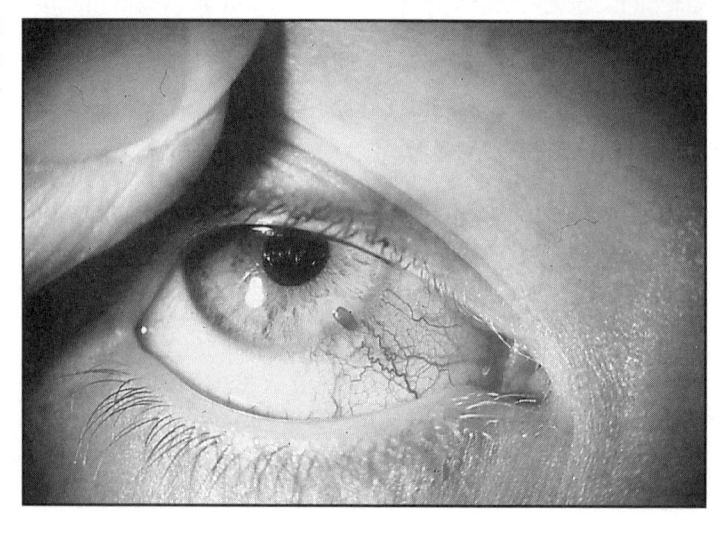

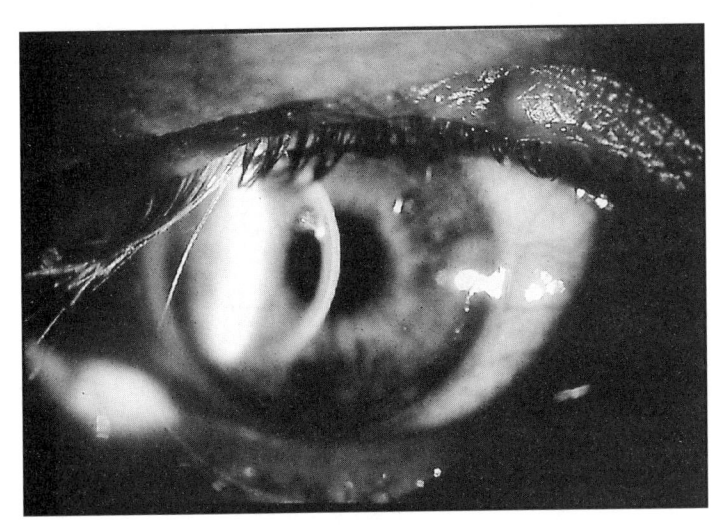

Figure 4-23. Corneal wood chip FB. (Photograph courtesy of EL Hargis, MD.)

A B-scan ultrasound may be used to determine if there is an intraocular FB, and a CT scan may be obtained to rule out an intraocular or intraorbital FB (see Chapter 8).

Document visual acuity before any treatment is given. Treatment includes applying a topical anesthetic and removing the foreign material(s). If there are multiple FBs, a saline rinse can be used to wash away the loose particles. Corneal FBs can be dislodged with use of topical anesthetics and an FB spud or a needle (Figure 4-24). If there is a rust ring, it can sometimes be removed with the spud, but this is usually done with a rust ring drill or burr that has a rotating head to help scour away the rust (Figure 4-25).

Surface conjunctival FBs can sometimes be removed with topical anesthetic and a cotton-tipped applicator or an FB spud. Embedded conjunctival FBs may need to be extracted with forceps.

After removal of corneal FBs, the resultant epithelial defect will be measured, a topical cycloplegic and antibiotic instilled, and a pressure patch applied for 24 hours. If the corneal defect was small and not centrally located, the patient may be instructed to remove the patch after 24 hours, use topical antibiotics for a few days, and return for follow up as needed. If the defect was large or centrally located, the patient will need to return for re-evaluation in 24 hours.

After removal of conjunctival FBs, topical antibiotics and artificial tears may be prescribed, with follow-up as needed.

Corneal Lacerations

Corneal lacerations may extend only partially into the cornea (Figure 4-26), or may be through the entire thickness of the cornea (a penetrating injury) (Figures 4-27 and 4-28).

A partial thickness laceration will be carefully examined to rule out blood in the anterior chamber, to evaluate anterior chamber depth, and to establish that a perforation does not exist (by means of Seidel's test, described above). If the laceration is small, it may be treated as a corneal abrasion. If the laceration has a wound gap, it may be sutured in the operating room. Topical cycloplegics and antibiotics will be instilled and a pressure patch applied, or sometimes a bandage soft contact lens is used. The patient will be examined each day until the epithelium has healed.

A full thickness corneal laceration, in which the entire corneal thickness has been penetrated, may be small and show no aqueous leakage. In this case the wound may be treated with topical antibiotics and a light pressure patch or bandage soft contact lens. Larger lacerations with aque-

Figure 4-24. FB spud. (Photograph courtesy of LS Sims, COT.)

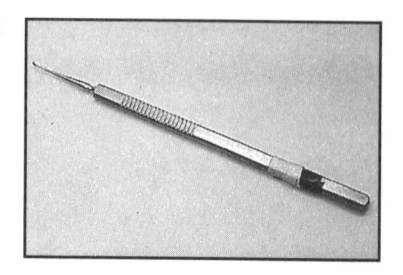

Figure 4-25. FB drill. (Photograph courtesy of LS Sims, COT.)

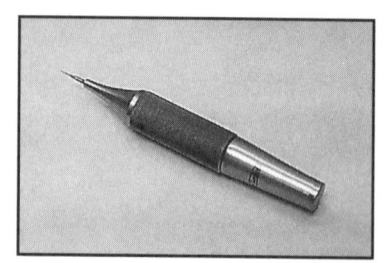

Figure 4-26. Partial corneal laceration. (Photograph courtesy of Paula Parker, COMT.)

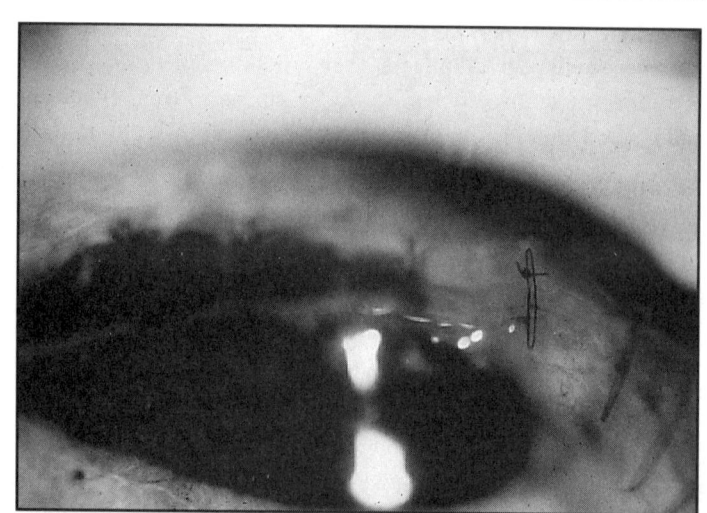

Figure 4-27. Corneal perforation plugged with blood and mucus. (Photograph courtesy of Paula Parker, COMT.)

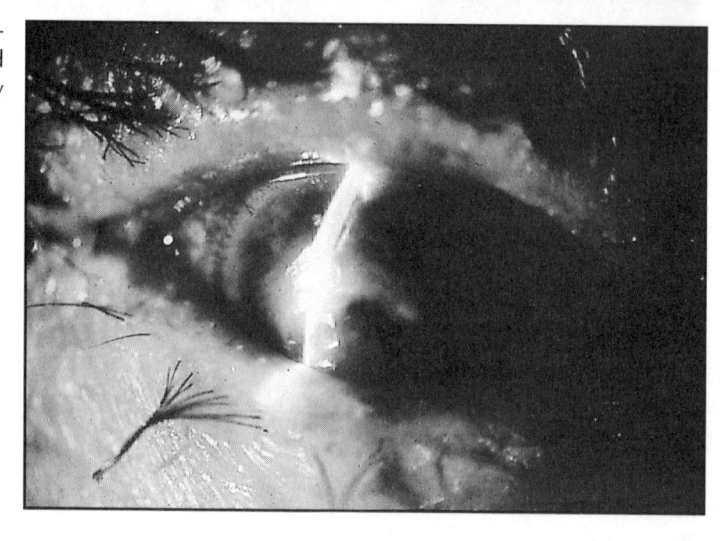

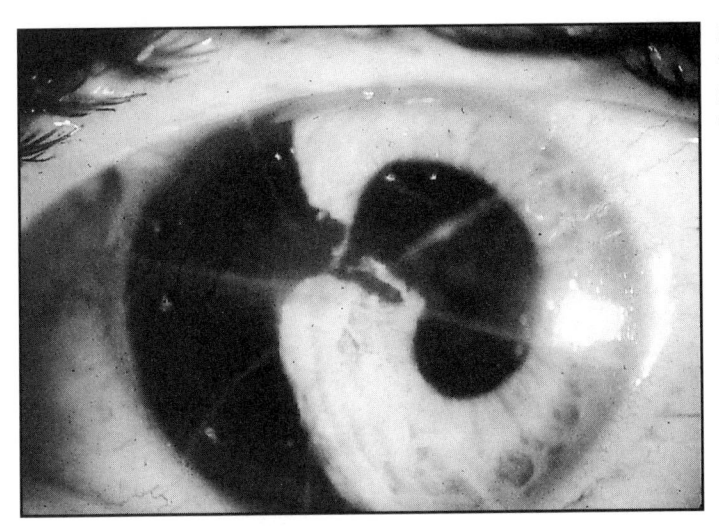

Figure 4-28. Ruptured cornea with iris involvement. (Photograph courtesy of Paula Parker, COMT.)

ous leakage may show signs of increased or decreased anterior chamber depth, an elevated or low IOP, and an irregular pupil. These usually require surgical repair. In any full thickness laceration, endophthalmitis is a concern (see Chapter 8).

Conjunctival Lacerations

A patient with a conjunctival laceration may report a recent ocular trauma and have symptoms of ocular pain (or an FB sensation) and redness. The tear in the conjunctival tissue and the exposed sclera can be seen with the use of fluorescein dye. There may also be a conjunctival or subconjunctival hemorrhage.

The eye will be examined to rule out a ruptured globe or a penetrating FB. CT scan and B-scan ultrasound may be performed to rule out intraocular or intraorbital FBs.

If the globe has not been ruptured, small wounds may be treated with an antibiotic ointment and a 24 hour pressure patch. Large wounds may require surgical repair.

Chapter 5

Emergencies and Injuries of the Lens

Leslie Hargis-Greenshields, COMT

KEY POINTS

- The crystalline lens is a transparent, biconvex, avascular structure suspended behind the iris by ligaments called zonules.
- A cataract is the most common result of injury to the lens.
- Age of onset, location of the opacity, stage of development, and etiology are methods of classifying cataracts.
- Trauma is the most common cause of an acquired dislocated lens.

Anatomy of the Lens

The crystalline lens is a transparent, biconvex, avascular, structure capable of changing shape. The lens lies posterior to the iris and anterior to the vitreous face, and is centered behind the pupil. The lens is held in place by zonules, which originate in the ciliary body and insert into the lens equator (Figure 5-1).

It is the change in shape or convexity of the lens that allows the eye to focus up close (or *accommodate*). Unlike other structures in the body, the lens continues to grow throughout life. Over the years, the lens gradually loses its elasticity due to the compression of the mature fibers in the central nucleus. Presbyopia is the loss of accommodative ability due to this decrease in lens elasticity.

Since the lens is an avascular tissue, there are no nerves, pain sensors, or lymphatic channels. For this reason there are no tumors or infections of the lens itself. There are really only two types of injuries that affect the lens. They are a change in lens position and cataracts.

Lenticular Dislocations

Ectopia Lentis

Ectopia lentis refers to a displacement of the lens. This may be either a total or a partial displacement. Trauma is the most common cause of an acquired lens dislocation, especially in childhood (where it can be associated with child abuse). Typically, blunt trauma tears the zonules that hold the lens in place behind the iris. A complete rupture of the zonules results in a free-floating or totally displaced lens. A partial severance of the zonules results in a partially dislocated (subluxated) lens.

Two common signs of a displaced lens are iridodonesis and phacodonesis. Iridodonesis is a quivering of the iris upon movement of the eye. This results from the lack of normal support of the lens. Phacodonesis is a wobbling of the lens upon movement of the eye. This is due to lack of support from the zonules. Other ocular findings associated with a displaced lens include non-corneal astigmatism, cataracts, and occasionally the presence of vitreous in the anterior chamber. Complications of a displaced lens include refractive problems, pupillary block glaucoma, and lenticular/corneal touch. Symptoms of a displaced lens include fluctuating or decreased vision, glare, and monocular diplopia. However, unless a cataract forms or the patient's vision is impaired the condition is usually left untreated.

Total Dislocation

The lens may be completely displaced from its normal position (centered behind the pupil). This is referred to as a luxation or total dislocation of the lens. The lens is moved away from the pupillary area and may fall forward into the anterior chamber or posteriorly into the vitreous (Figure 5-2).

Dislocation of the lens into the anterior chamber may cause pupillary block and angle-closure glaucoma with other secondary complications, such as iritis. The anteriorly-displaced lens may also cause damage to the endothelial cells due to lenticular/corneal touch. Treatment is surgical removal of the lens. Dislocation of the lens into the vitreous often causes no secondary complications, so it is not treated either medically or surgically.

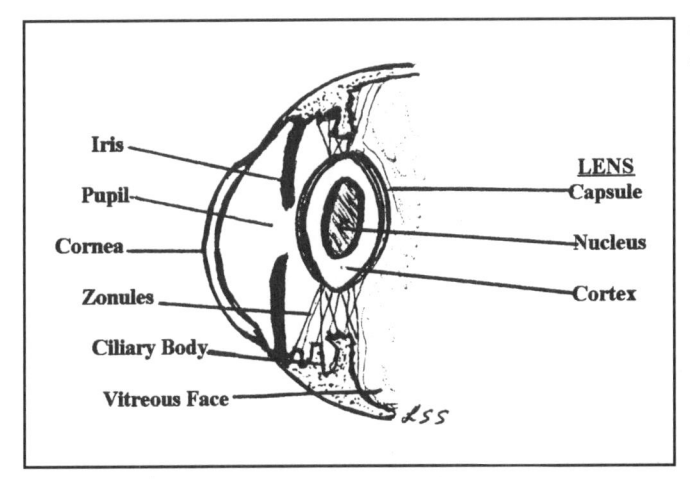

Figure 5-1. Schematic of lens anatomy. (Illustration courtesy of LS Sims, COT.)

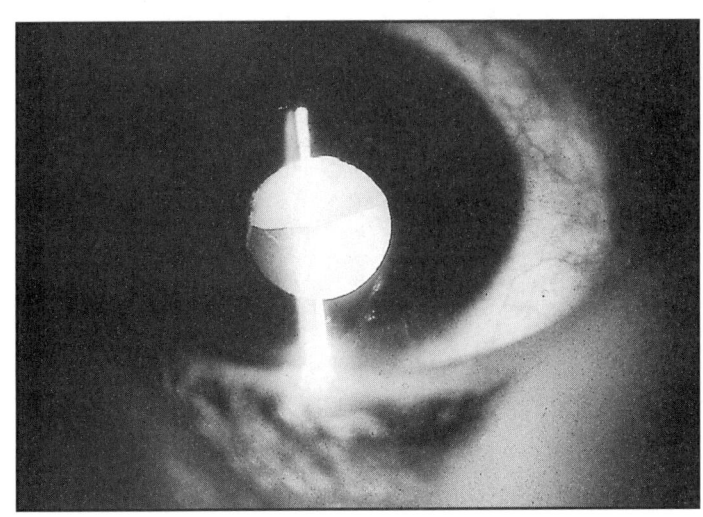

Figure 5-2. Dislocated lens. (Photograph courtesy of Paula Parker, COMT.)

Subluxation

The lens may be partially dislocated or subluxated from its normal position. In this situation, the lens is pulled towards the zonules that remain intact. The lens is moved out of its centered position behind the iris but remains in the pupillary area (Figure 5-3).

The main complications of a partially displaced lens are decreased or distorted vision, glaucoma, and uveitis. Treatment of a partially displaced lens is required only if the symptoms are visually disabling or if complications develop.

Treatment may include:
- Glasses—to correct for induced astigmatism or aphakia
- Lasering of zonules—to move the lens out of the visual axis
- Lens extraction—for lens-induced glaucoma and uveitis

Patients with a dislocated lens as a result of a traumatic injury should also be evaluated for other signs of ocular injury. Patients with a dislocated lens may remain asymptomatic for years; however, they should still be warned of the signs associated with pupillary block glaucoma. These patients should also be encouraged to wear protective eyewear during sports and other hazardous situations.

Figure 5-3. Subluxated lens. (Photograph courtesy of Leslie Hargis-Greenshields, COMT.)

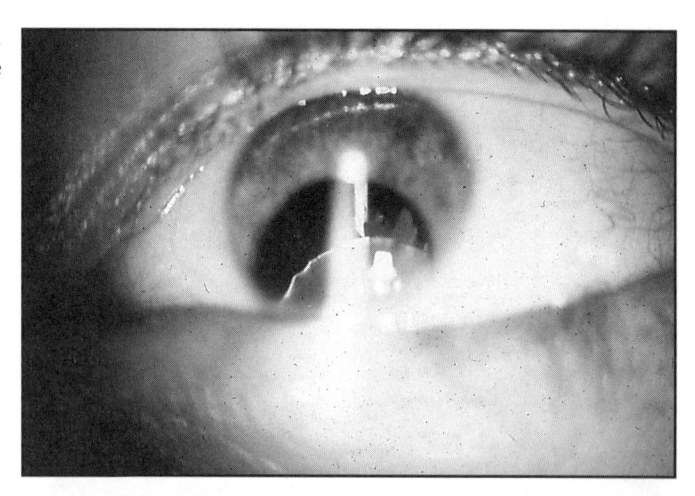

Figure 5-4. Intraocular lens implant (IOL). (Photograph courtesy of Paula Parker, COMT.)

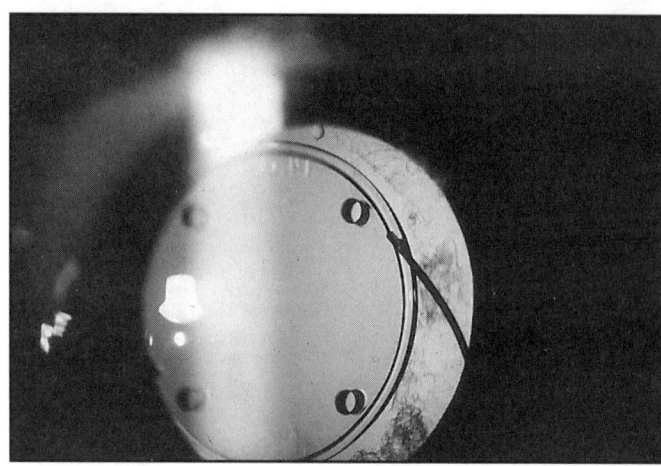

Cataracts

A cataract is any opacity of the lens; it is not a growth. The usual cause for cataracts is age, although they can be caused by injury ("traumatic cataract"). The only treatment for a cataract is to remove it (ie, remove the entire lens). When the lens is removed, much of the focusing power of the eye goes with it. This is replaced by inserting an intraocular lens (IOL) implant at the time of surgery (Figure 5-4). For more detailed information about cataracts, please consult Basic Bookshelf title *Cataract and Glaucoma for the Eyecare Paraprofessional*.

It is important to note that if trauma results in a cataract during childhood, amblyopia may develop. The cataract acts as an occluder, preventing the development of the visual pathway in that eye.

Classifications

One of the methods used to describe, and therefore classify, an opacification of the lens is according to the age at onset. Congenital, infantile, juvenile, adult, and senile are the categories used in this method of classification. This category is not typically used in describing trauma or emergencies of the lens, since trauma can occur at any age.

Cataracts can also be classified according to where in the lens the cataract is located. This could be nuclear, cortical, capsular, or subcapsular. The location of a traumatic cataract depends on the type of trauma and the extent of injury. Blunt trauma usually causes opacities in the anterior or posterior subcapsular area. An injury that penetrates the lens capsule produces hydration of the lens protein, causing a dense white cortical cataract. Ionizing radiation may cause fine anterior subcapsular opacities. If the opacity is not in the optic zone and/or is not interfering with the patient's vision, it is often left untreated.

Cataracts may also be described according to their stage of development. How quickly a cataract forms depends on whether the lens capsule was ruptured. If the capsule was not ruptured, a cataract may not develop for months following the original trauma. If the capsule was ruptured, the lens may become hydrated and form a cataract within hours. Not all cataracts are progressive; a small rent in the lens may seal itself by forming fibrous cortical tissue at the site of injury.

The following is a list of cataracts classified by developmental stage:
- Immature—a mild, asymptomatic cataract where the opacities are separated by clear areas (Figure 5-5)
- Intumescent—swollen with water; can be immature or mature
- Mature—has a cortex that is entirely white and opaque (Figure 5-6)
- Hypermature—has become smaller with a wrinkled capsule as water leaks out of the lens
- Morgagnian—a hypermature cataract where the cortical fibers have liquefied and allowed the nucleus to drop inferiorly in the bag.

The typical classifications of cataracts according to maturity or stage of development are not particularly helpful in describing traumatic cataracts. The later stages of cataract development may lead to an angle-closure attack or lens-induced glaucoma, both of which could cause an ocular emergency.

Traumatic Cataracts

Trauma is the most common cause of unilateral cataracts (Figures 5-7 and 5-8). A traumatic cataract may be the lens's response to contusion, concussion, laceration, intraocular FB, or radiation.

A *contusion* injury is the result of a direct blow to the eye that causes the lens capsule to rupture. The resulting cataract is star-shaped and is typically located in the posterior lens.

A *concussion* injury occurs when the force of a blow (not striking the eye) causes damage via tissue conduction or air conduction of that force. A head injury is a common cause of concussion injury to the eye through tissue conduction. In this case, a blow to the head causes waves of the force to be conducted to the eye through tissue (ie, bone and orbital fat). An explosion is an example of a concussion injury conducted by air; the waves hit the cornea and are transmitted to the ocular structures, causing injury to the eyeball. Either type of conduction can cause injury to the crystalline lens, resulting in cataract formation. Although not a cataract per se, a concussive injury may also cause the iris to be pushed against the lens momentarily. This can leave an "imprint" of iris pigment, known as a Vossius' ring, on the anterior lens surface. The pigment may disappear with time.

Any *lacerating* or penetrating injury to the anterior segment may be complicated by injury to the crystalline lens. Damage to the lens can vary from a small rent in the capsule causing a tiny localized cataract, to complete disruption with lens material filling the anterior chamber. This dispersion of lens material may produce a uveitis and/or a secondary glaucoma. With any penetrating injury, other ocular trauma and complications should be ruled out.

Figure 5-5. Immature cataract. (Photograph courtesy of Paula Parker, COMT.)

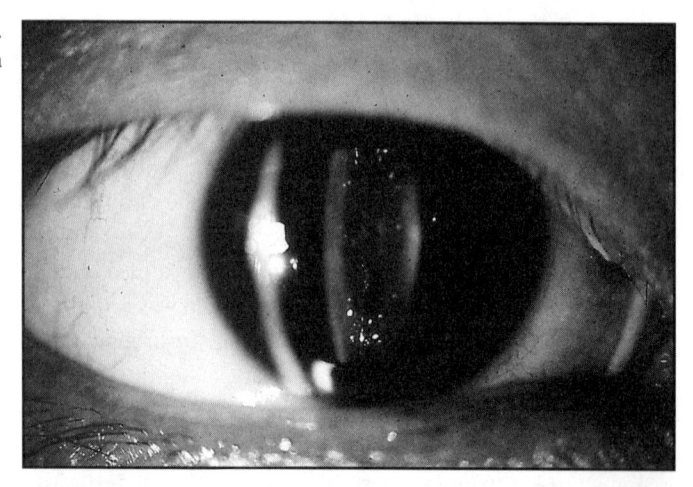

Figure 5-6. Mature cataract. (Photograph courtesy of Leslie Hargis-Greenshields, COMT.)

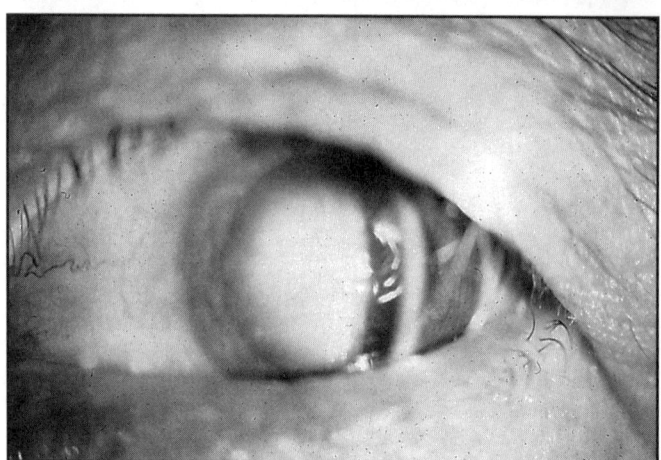

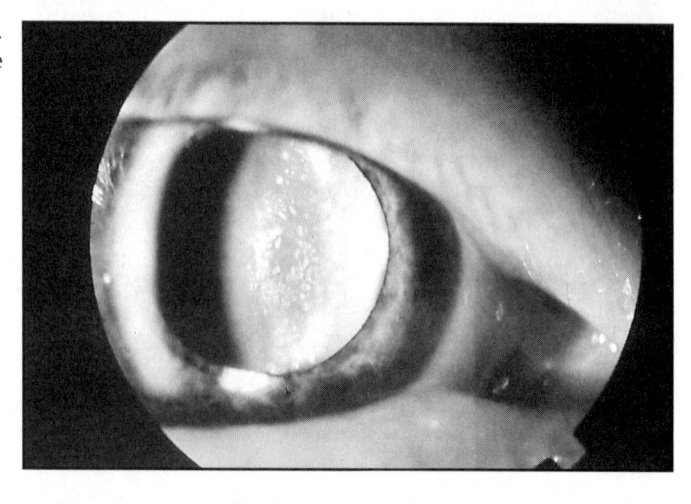

Figure 5-7. Traumatic cataract. (Photograph courtesy of Leslie Hargis-Greenshields, COMT.)

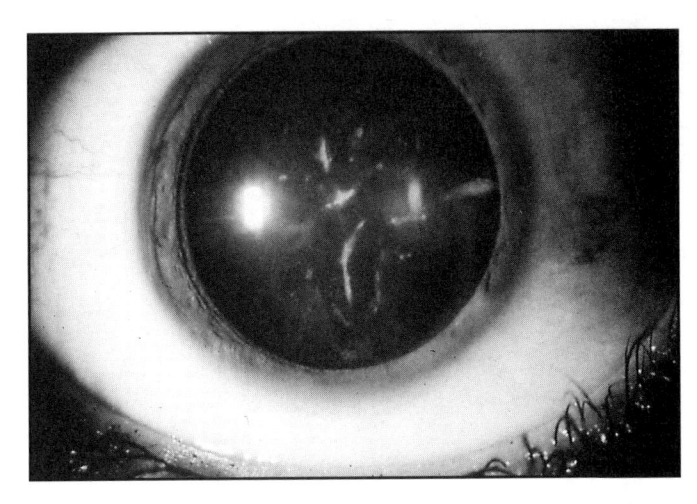

Figure 5-8. Traumatic cataract. (Photograph courtesy of TD Lindquist, MD, PhD.)

The eye reacts to an *intraocular FB* in different ways, depending on the FB. The FB also reacts differently in different ocular tissues. Typically, an FB in the anterior chamber or in the lens causes much less of a reaction than an FB in the retina. The injury caused by an FB is also determined by its size, composition, and momentum. A metallic FB may cause toxic damage to the lens as the metal is oxidized, causing a cataract. A copper particle generally causes a sunflower-shaped cataract known as chalcosis lentis. An iron particle may cause a rusty brown or yellow colored cataract known as siderosis lentis.

Several types of trauma fall into the category of *electromagnetic radiation*. Infrared (or heat waves), electric shock, and ionizing radiation are the most common causes of cataracts, although there are others. Infrared damage is described as a "glassblower's cataract." This type of cataract was common in industries where workers were exposed to infrared radiation for prolonged periods and was more prevalent before the development of protective eyewear. Cataracts from electric shock (including lightning strikes) are seen in anywhere from 5% to 20% of shock cases. Most develop some kind of opacification within the first 12 months after the injury, especially if the voltage was higher than 1,000. The entrance wounds are typically on the head and neck.

The eye is extremely sensitive to *ionizing radiation*, which may be used to treat ocular or brain tumors. Depending on the dose of radiation, there may be a latent period of up to 20 years before a cataract appears. The younger eye tends to be more susceptible to such damage. Radiation cataracts from exposure to X-rays are sometimes seen in infants whose mothers were exposed to X-rays during the first 3 months of pregnancy.

Severe cold can also trigger the onset of a traumatic cataract.

Chapter 6

Glaucoma

Leslie Hargis-Greenshields, COMT

KEY POINTS

- Glaucoma can be classified into two major categories: primary glaucoma and secondary glaucoma.

- Primary glaucoma implies a separate disease process unrelated to any other ocular or systemic condition.

- Secondary glaucoma is the consequence of another recognizable ocular or orbital disease, systemic disorder, or other cause.

- The acute angle-closure glaucoma patient tends to be seen on an emergent basis due to his or her sudden onset of symptoms.

- An acute glaucoma attack can be characterized by severe pain around the eye, decreased vision due to a hazy cornea, mid-dilated pupil, and gastrointestinal symptoms such as nausea and vomiting.

Introduction

Glaucoma is defined as an increase in IOP significant enough to cause damage to the optic nerve and visual field. The increase in IOP is the result of either a mechanical blockage of the flow of aqueous within the eye or a decrease in the volume of aqueous drainage from the eye.

Aqueous humor is produced in the ciliary body and flows from the posterior chamber, through the pupil, into the anterior chamber, (where it drains through the trabecular meshwork and Schlemm's canal) and is then absorbed into the venous system (Figure 6-1). Glaucoma can be classified into two major categories: primary glaucoma and secondary glaucoma. For a complete discussion of glaucoma, please see Basic Bookshelf title *Cataract and Glaucoma for the Eyecare Paraprofessional*.

Primary Glaucoma

Primary glaucoma suggests a separate disease process unrelated to any other ocular or systemic condition. Primary glaucoma may be further broken down into open-angle glaucoma and angle-closure glaucoma.

Primary Open-Angle Glaucoma

In open-angle glaucoma, the aqueous humor has unrestricted access to the trabecular meshwork, or drainage system, of the eye, yet drainage is not adequate. Primary open-angle glaucoma (POAG) is the most common form of glaucoma. Careful patient questioning may uncover a familial history of this disease. Its onset is usually gradual and asymptomatic, and is frequently revealed when tonometry shows an increase in the IOP. Visual acuity is not usually affected until later in the disease process. The loss of vision can be documented and followed by comparisons of repeated visual field tests. Optic disk changes are the most important early findings. Careful ophthalmoscopic examination by the physician may find a disparity in the cup size between the two eyes. Other changes of the optic disk involve vertical enlargement of the cup, erosion of the rim, disk hemorrhages, bending of the vessels at the margin, and (finally) total cupping of the entire disk. Treatment of POAG begins with medications, then laser, and finally surgical intervention if there is no success in lowering IOP with the previous treatments. Since POAG is not typically related to an emergent situation, we will not spend any more time on this category.

Primary Angle-Closure Glaucoma

Primary angle-closure glaucoma (PACG) makes up less than 10% of the primary glaucomas. However, due to its sudden onset of symptoms, angle-closure glaucoma is frequently seen on an emergent basis. In angle-closure glaucoma there is a mechanical blockage somewhere along the pathway of aqueous production or flow, resulting in an increase in IOP. An acute attack of angle-closure glaucoma develops only in an eye that has an anatomically narrow angle (Figures 6-2 and 6-3). If there is contact between the iris and the anterior surface of the lens (such as a posterior synechia), the flow of aqueous is blocked from the posterior chamber to the anterior chamber (Figure 6-4). As pressure builds in the posterior chamber, the peripheral iris is pushed forward. If the iris is pushed far enough forward it may actually block the trabecular meshwork, causing an acute angle-closure glaucoma attack (Figure 6-5).

Glaucoma 55

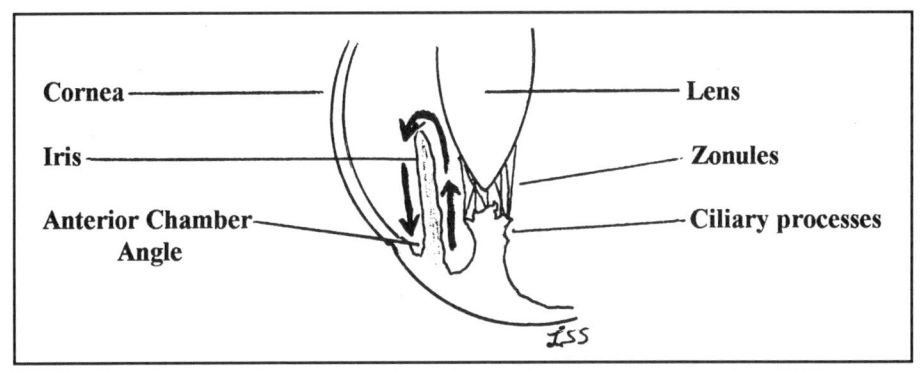

Figure 6-1. Schematic of aqueous outflow. (Illustration courtesy of LS Sims, COT.)

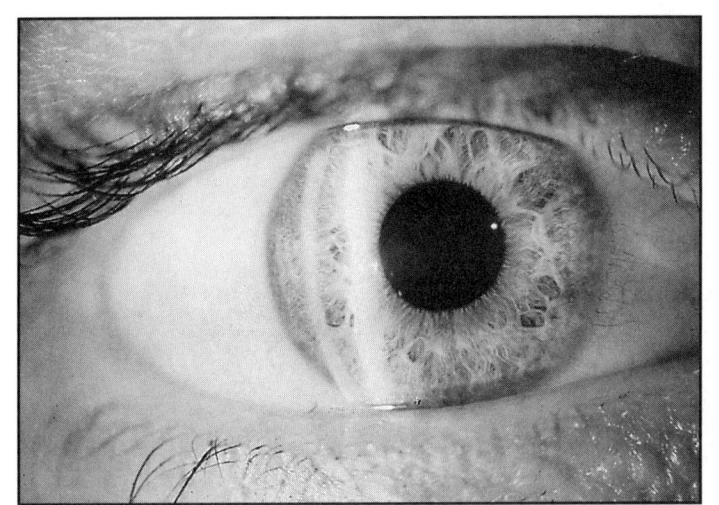

Figure 6-2. Open angle. (Photograph courtesy of Leslie Hargis-Greenshields, COMT.)

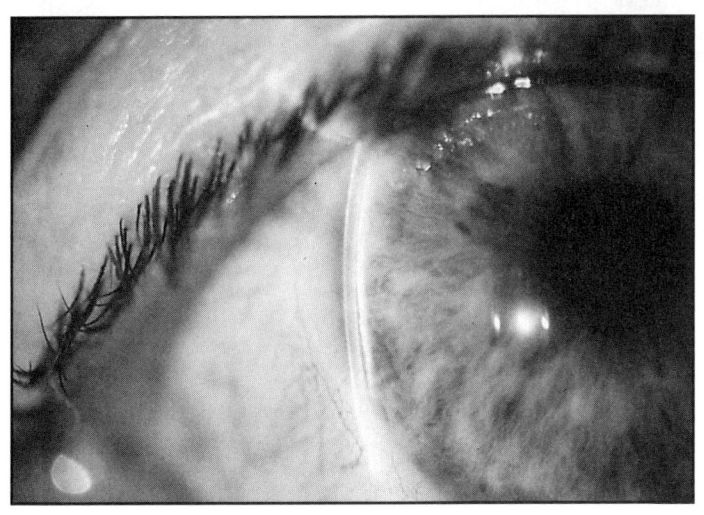

Figure 6-3. Narrow angle. (Photograph courtesy of Leslie Hargis-Greenshields, COMT.)

Figure 6-4. Posterior synechia. (Photograph courtesy of TD Lindquist, MD, PhD.)

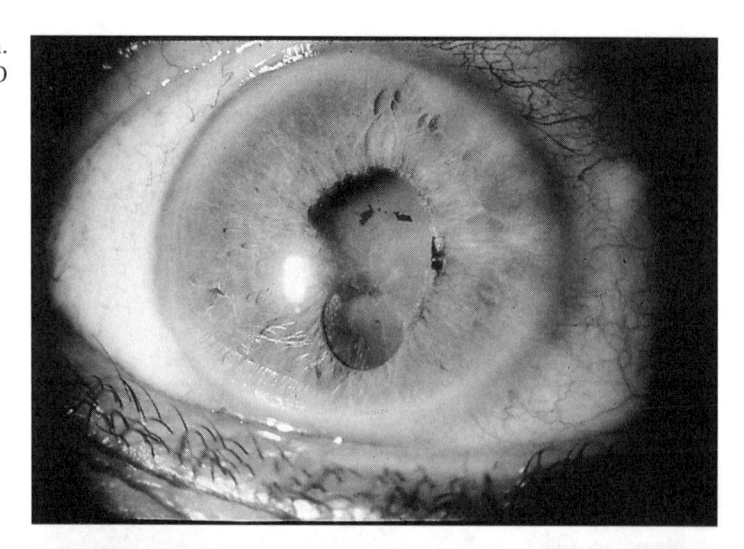

Figure 6-5. Angle-closure attack. (Photograph courtesy of TD Lindquist, MD, PhD.)

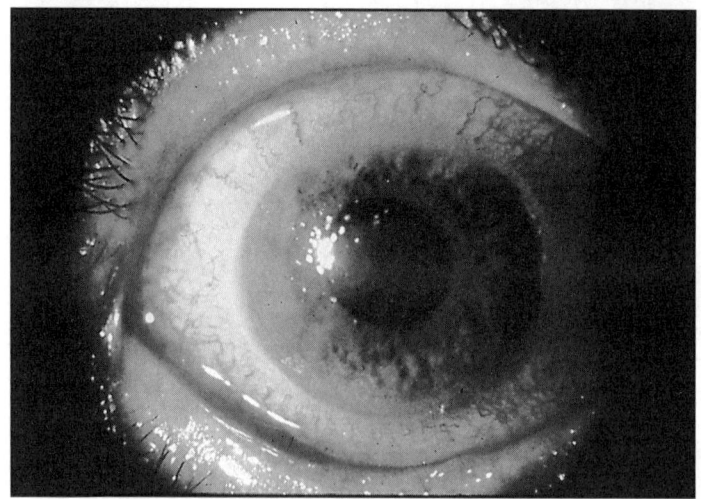

Typically, acute angle-closure glaucoma affects people over age 50 and its prevalence increases with age. It is four times more likely to occur in women than in men and is more common in certain races (such as persons of Northern European decent).

There are several inherited anatomic factors that predispose certain individuals to angle-closure glaucoma:
- A shallow anterior chamber
- A narrow entrance to the angle structures
- A short axial length
- An increased lens thickness
- A small corneal diameter

Dilating drops and certain antihistamines can precipitate an angle-closure attack in individuals with narrow angles. For the assistant using dilating drops it is important to check the status of the patient's angles prior to dilation. This can be done using a pen light or by the estimating the depth of the anterior chamber at the slit lamp. If the angles appear narrow, ask your doctor to see if they may occlude before you instill dilating medication.

Ocular findings of PACG include a markedly increased IOP, ciliary flush, tearing, photophobia, corneal edema, shallow anterior chamber, and a mid-dilated pupil. Other symptoms may include a sudden onset of blurred vision followed by a dull throbbing pain in and around the eye. The patient may describe rainbows or halos around light sources due to the corneal edema. Gastrointestinal symptoms such as nausea and vomiting are not uncommon.

Treatment of PACG starts with medical intervention to reduce the IOP. This is done by both systemic and topical medications including hyperosmotic agents, carbonic anhydrase inhibitors, beta-blockers, and miotics. A peripheral laser iridotomy is done after the pressure has been brought under control to re-establish the flow of aqueous between the posterior and anterior chambers. Finally, surgical treatment in the form of a filtering procedure is done if the eye failed to respond to the iridotomy.

Secondary Glaucoma*

Secondary glaucoma occurs as the result of another ocular or systemic disease. Any history of previous eye surgery, inflammation, or injury to an eye, combined with pain, redness, and blurred vision may indicate a secondary angle-closure attack. Sometimes these occurrences can happen months or even years after the initial injury or surgery.

Since there are many ocular conditions that can cause secondary glaucoma, it is difficult to classify. However, one way to classify the secondary glaucomas is to separate them into two major categories: open-angle and angle-closure. We can also distinguish the secondary glaucomas into types that obstruct the trabecular meshwork, those that are lens-induced (or related), or those that result from complications of other trauma.

Typically, patients will appear in the office or emergency room with secondary glaucoma because of the symptoms associated with an angle-closure attack. The treatments of secondary glaucoma are about as varied as the situation themselves. For the most part, treatment is divided into two categories: treatment of the elevated IOP and treatment of the causative disease.

The information in this section is not listed in the criteria for the ophthalmic technician exam.

Obstructed Trabeculum

Acute Anterior Uveitis

In early uveitis the IOP is frequently normal or lower than normal because the inflamed ciliary body is not functioning properly. Occasionally, a trabecular block develops, secondarily obstructing the aqueous outflow with inflammatory cells or debris. The IOP typically returns to normal once the inflammation has cleared.

Chronic Anterior Uveitis

In chronic or long standing uveitis the outflow facility is restricted by anterior synechiae or trabecular scarring. Treatment is typically the prevention of synechiae through the use of topical and injectable steroids, the lowering of IOP through the use of topical and/or systemic medications, and an iridotomy if the medical treatment was not successful.

Hemolytic Glaucoma

Hemolytic glaucoma is another mechanical obstruction of the trabecular meshwork which can occur following trauma. A hyphema is bleeding in the anterior chamber as the result of a tear

Figure 6-6. Hyphema. (Photograph courtesy of Paula Parker, COMT.)

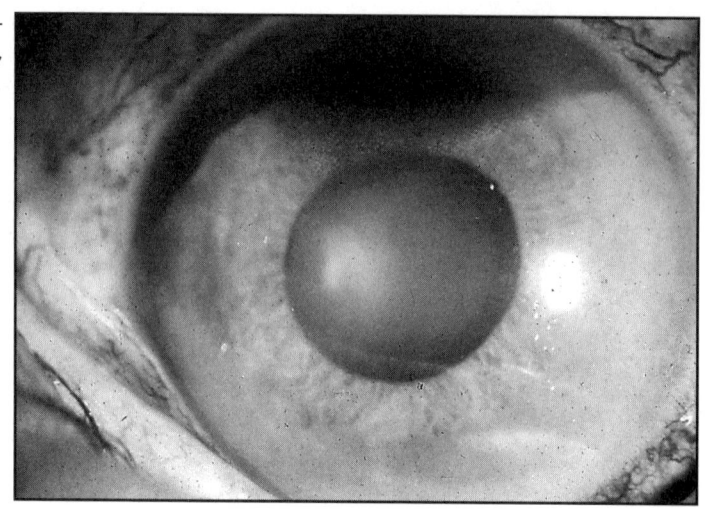

or injury to the iris or ciliary body. In hemolytic glaucoma, the elevation of IOP is caused by blockage of the trabeculum with red blood cells (Figure 6-6). In some cases a blood clot may block the pupil, resulting in an angle-closure aspect to this type of injury.

The treatment of a secondary hemolytic glaucoma is either medical or surgical. Treatment with medication depends on the level of IOP. Surgical treatment may be required to remove the blood from the anterior chamber, depending on the degree of blood and level of IOP.

Ghost Cell Glaucoma

Ghost cell glaucoma occurs as a result of a vitreous hemorrhage. Frequently it is seen in blunt trauma or surgery where the anterior face of the vitreous is ruptured and blood from a vitreous hemorrhage enters the anterior segment. Ghost cells are denatured red blood cells that become trapped in the trabecular meshwork causing an obstruction in the outflow of aqueous. The increase in IOP is dependent on the number of ghost cells entering the anterior chamber.

Treatment is typically medical. If medications are unsuccessful then the surgeon may irrigate the anterior chamber to wash out the ghost cells.

Traumatic Angle Recession

Traumatic angle recession is the result of blunt trauma which tears the anterior face of the ciliary body. Glaucoma may not develop until months or even years after the initial injury. The exact mechanism of this glaucoma is not known. Current thought is that the increase in IOP is due to damage to the trabeculum rather than from the angle recession itself. Typically, the larger the area of recession, the higher the risk of developing glaucoma.

Treatment is the same for other types of open-angle glaucoma, with the exception that miotics aren't used.

Epithelial Ingrowth

Epithelial ingrowth from the site of a previous surgical incision is caused by an invasion of epithelial cells into the anterior chamber through a defect in the surgical incision. This can cause obstruction of the aqueous flow at the angle of the anterior chamber.

Treatment consists of cryotherapy to destroy the epithelial cells on the ciliary body and endothelium. The membrane may be removed with a vitreous cutter.

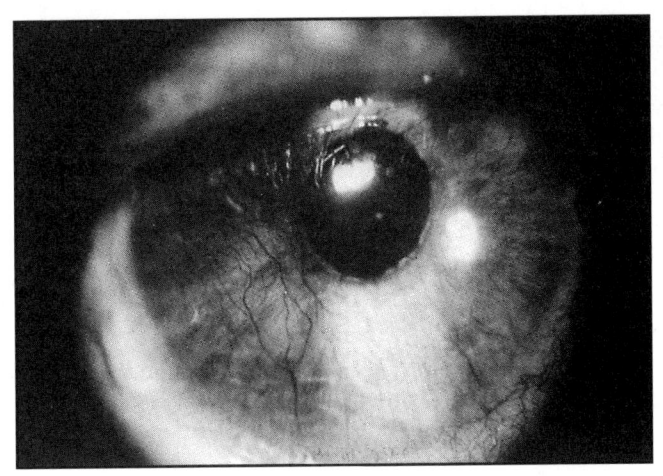

Figure 6-7. Iris neovascularization (rubeosis). (Reprinted with permission from Herrin M. *Ophthalmic Examination and Basic Skills.* Thorofare, NJ: SLACK Incorporated; 1990.)

Neovascular Glaucoma

In neovascular glaucoma, the increased IOP is caused by actual closure of the angle through contraction of fibrous vascular tissue. In the early stage of neovascular glaucoma, new abnormal blood vessels grow radially over the iris surface (rubeosis iridis) towards the angle (Figure 6-7). In the final stages of secondary angle-closure glaucoma, the fibrous vascular tissue that has grown into the angle contracts, pulling the peripheral iris over the trabeculum.

Treatment is varied and includes panretinal photocoagulation (PRP), retinal surgery, medical therapy, and artificial filtering shunts. The goal of treatment in final stages of neovascular glaucoma is primarily to relieve pain. This may be done by a retrobulbar alcohol injection or enucleation (if all other treatments fail).

Lens-Related Secondary Glaucomas

Phacolytic Glaucoma

Phacolytic glaucoma is a secondary open-angle glaucoma that occurs when a hypermature lens cortex liquifies and leaks through the lens capsule. The trabecular meshwork is obstructed with lens proteins and macrophages, causing an increase in IOP. The patient presents with a hypermature cataract and white particles in the aqueous. Treatment includes lowering the IOP with medications, followed by removal of the cataract.

Lens Particle Glaucoma

Lens particle glaucoma occurs when there is an incomplete removal of the lens material during cataract surgery or as a result of lens particles being released into the eye following trauma. White fluffy remnants of lens cortex are seen in the pupillary opening and over the trabecular meshwork, causing an elevation in IOP. Treatment is the same as with phacolytic glaucoma.

Phacomorphic Glaucoma

Phacomorphic glaucoma occurs when in intumescent or swollen cataractous lens pushes against the back of the iris causing pupillary block and a secondary angle-closure. Treatment starts with the medicinal lowering of the IOP. Once the pressure is controlled, a laser iridotomy is performed and finally the cataract is removed.

Lens Dislocation

A lens dislocated into the anterior chamber as a result of blunt trauma can cause a rapid increase in IOP due to pupillary block. Urgent surgical treatment is required, as lens/cornea contact will cause permanent damage to the endothelium.

Other Traumatic Secondary Glaucomas

Chemical Burns

Alkalis (bases) can quickly penetrate the cornea and anterior chamber causing extensive damage. Penetrating alkalis soften tissue by disrupting living cells. Complicated cataracts and/or secondary glaucoma are common after chemical injuries. The first order of treatment is to control the damage of the chemical burn and then address each area of complication separately.

Chapter 7

Emergencies and Injuries of the Uveal Tract

Janice K. (Jan) Ledford, COMT

KEY POINTS

- The uveal tract consists of the iris, the ciliary body, and the choroid.
- Uveitis refers to inflammation of the uvea. It can be further identified by citing which part of the uvea is involved.
- Uveitis can be precipitated by trauma (injury or surgery) or linked to an inflammatory process in the body as a whole.
- The effects of blunt trauma to the uvea can include: traumatic iritis, recessed angle, Vossius' ring, iridodialysis, hyphema, and choroidal hemorrhage.
- If the sclera is lacerated, uveal material may exude (prolapse) through the wound.
- Where there has been a penetrating injury (accidental or surgical) to one eye, the uninjured eye may be at risk for developing sympathetic ophthalmia. The injured eye develops a uveitis, then the uninjured eye begins to "sympathize" with its fellow. The result is a bilateral panuveitis.

Anatomy of the Uveal Tract

The uveal tract is made up of three structures: the iris, the ciliary body, and the choroid. These structures are highly vascular and are an important source of blood to the retina and other structures.

The iris is the most anterior part of the uvea. It is comprised of the sphincter and dilator muscles. These muscles control the size of the pupil, and thus the amount of light entering the eye. Anterior to the iris is the anterior chamber. The posterior chamber lies behind the iris and extends to the vitreous humor. (Both the anterior and posterior chambers comprise the anterior *segment* of the eye.) The back surface of the iris is pigmented.

The ciliary body serves to connect the iris and choroid. It is a roughly triangle-shaped structure that extends from the anterior part of the choroid to the root of the iris. The ciliary body has two zones. The most forward zone is the pars plicata, which is a pleated structure. The posterior zone is the pars plana, which has a smooth surface. The ciliary processes and their overlying epithelium, which form the aqueous humor, originate in the pars plicata. The ciliary muscle is also part of the ciliary body. This muscle serves to control accommodation (focusing of the lens).

The choroid, which comprises the largest part of the uvea, lies between the retina and sclera. It is firmly anchored into the edges of the optic nerve at the back of the eye, and extends forward to merge with the ciliary body. The choroid is highly pigmented due to the presence of melanocytes scattered throughout the tissue. It contains a network of blood vessels that nourish the retina and sclera.

Uveitis

The term *uveitis* refers to inflammation of the uvea. It can be further identified by citing which part of the uvea is involved: the iris (iritis), the ciliary body (cyclitis), both the iris and ciliary body (iridocyclitis), or the choroid (choroiditis). Generally, however, the terms iritis and uveitis are used.

Anterior (Iritis)

Inflammation of the iris (iritis) can be precipitated by trauma (injury or surgery) or linked to an inflammatory process in the body as a whole (such as sarcoidosis or tuberculosis). It can also occur following an angle-closure glaucoma attack.

The patient will usually call or visit the office because of the pain and photophobia associated with iritis (Figure 7-1). Because iritis is accompanied by ocular redness, it is an important entity in the differential diagnosis of the red eye (see Chapter 9). It is important to note that the injection found in iritis is usually centralized around the limbus (versus the general redness of conjunctivitis or angle-closure glaucoma). In addition, there is no mucus discharge (versus that found in conjunctivitis), although there may be reflex tearing from the pain and photophobia. Finally, the pupil in an eye with iritis tends to be somewhat constricted, smaller than that of the fellow eye. (Conjunctivitis does not affect pupil size; in angle-closure glaucoma, the pupil is mid-dilated.) Vision is generally unaffected by iritis in its early stages, but may decrease thereafter. (Vision in conjunctivitis is basically normal unless there is mucus in the tear film. In angle-closure glaucoma, vision is decreased due to corneal edema.) These factors can be important in triage, especially via the phone. Acute iritis is an urgent situation, to be seen the same day. (Angle-closure glaucoma, on the other hand, is an emergency.)

Whatever the cause, the inflamed iris releases cells and debris into the aqueous. This can be

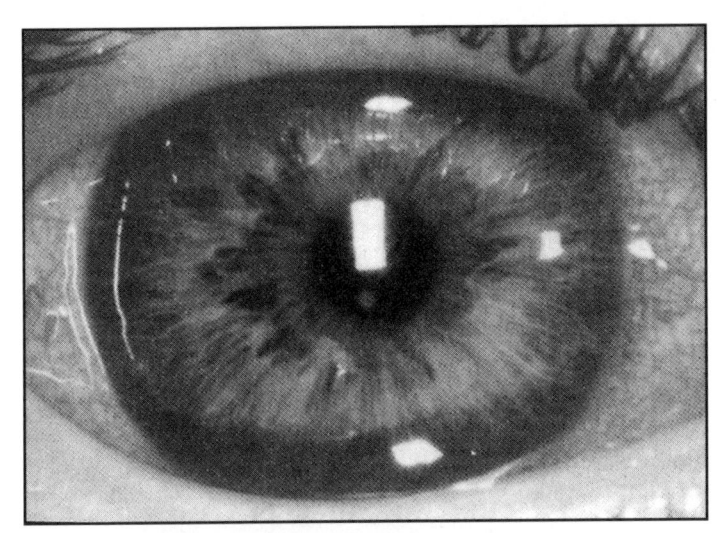

Figure 7-1. Iritis. (Reprinted with permission from Nemeth SC, Shea CA. *Medical Sciences for the Ophthalmic Assistant.* Thorofare, NJ: SLACK Incorporated; 1991.)

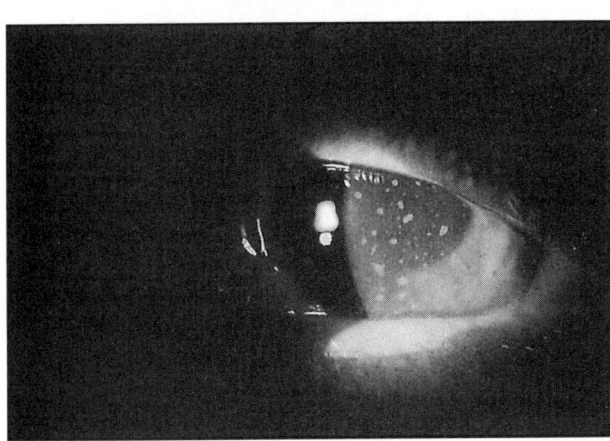

Figure 7-2. Keratitic precipitates. (Photo by Val Sanders. Reprinted with permission from Ledford JK, Sanders VN. *The Slit Lamp Primer.* Thorofare, NJ: SLACK Incorporated; 1998.)

seen on slit lamp examination as cells and flare in the anterior chamber. The floating material may congregate into clumps on the back surface of the cornea (keratitic precipitates, or KP's) (Figure 7-2). If the debris gets into the trabecular meshwork and impedes the outflow of aqueous, a secondary glaucoma can set up. The iris may form adhesions to the cornea (anterior synechia) or lens (posterior synechia).

Iritis is usually treated with topical steroids, and if the inflammation is severe, oral steroids may also be prescribed. Dilating drops are usually given as well, which help to reduce the patient's pain by keeping the iris still (much like putting a splint on a sprained wrist). The underlying cause of the iritis, if identified, may also be treated.

Posterior (Uveitis)

Posterior uveitis is usually referred to simply as uveitis. Like iritis, it can be associated with trauma (injury, especially penetrating, or surgery) or a systemic inflammatory process. Such inflammatory disorders include herpes zoster (shingles), herpes simplex (especially ocular), toxoplasmosis, histoplasmosis, rheumatoid arthritis, ankylosing spondylitis, sarcoidosis, tuberculosis, and chronic bowel disease. There are many types and causes of uveitis, so the best we can do here is offer general information.

The symptoms of uveitis include pain, redness, blurred vision, and photophobia. Onset may be sudden or gradual, and one or both eyes may be affected. If the inflammation is severe enough, synechiae, cataracts, macular edema, corneal edema, secondary glaucoma, and RD may occur.

Topical steroids (drops or ointment) are used to treat uveitis. Oral or injected steroids may be used as well. Sometimes NSAIDs are used. Dilating drops may be prescribed. If the cause of the uveitis is known, that will also be treated. In some cases, recovery occurs after a few days or weeks. In others, the inflammation seems to linger. Recurrence is common.

Blunt Trauma

Any trauma, blunt or otherwise, where there is decreased vision and/or pain should be considered an emergency. However, sometimes very severe trauma can be surprisingly asymptomatic, so it is always wise to err on the side of caution.

Iris

The mildest effect of blunt trauma to the eye is traumatic iritis. Its symptoms and treatment are basically the same as any anterior uveitis. Accommodative spasms may also occur after such an injury. To tell the difference between traumatic and medicinal mydriasis, the physician may instill a drop of 2% pilocarpine into the affected eye. This will cause a traumatic mydriasis to constrict promptly.

Blunt force to the eye may push the iris against the lens. The pressure of the compressed chamber may force aqueous into the ciliary body, causing a displacement of the trabecular tissue (a recessed angle). The recession may be so mild as to miss detection, or it may extend all the way back to the ciliary body. A hyphema usually accompanies a recessed angle. If the trabeculum is damaged severely enough, secondary glaucoma may develop. Not counting the sudden rise in IOP that occurs during the traumatic event itself, a later ocular hypertension may develop anywhere from 2 months to 2 years after the trauma, or even 10 to 15 years later.

If the iris is compacted against other structures in the eye it may leave pigment at points of contact, such as the corneal endothelium (usually at the angle) or the anterior lens capsule (known as Vossius' ring). Such trauma may also result in bleeding from the ciliary body, evident as a hyphema.

The weakest part of the iris is the root where the iris joins the ciliary body. If the traumatic force is enough to rip the iris (or part of it) from its root, the condition is called *iridodialysis*. This creates an "extra" pupil, as a hole exists where the iris is torn. The edge of the natural pupil is often flattened opposite the tear (a "D-shaped" pupil). Because iridodialysis occurs with severe trauma, it is likely that other ocular trauma has occurred as well. Traumatic iritis often develops and must be treated. The "extra" pupil may cause a disturbance in the patient's vision, most notably diplopia. If the diplopia is a continuing problem after healing, surgery may be needed to reattach the iris.

Iridodonesis is a condition where the iris shakes when the eye is moved. It is actually due to a dislocation of the lens, and is not specifically an iris injury.

Hyphema

Bleeding into the anterior chamber (hyphema) usually results from trauma (injury or surgery) or may be due to a blood clotting disorder (although this is rare). Signs and symptoms include a

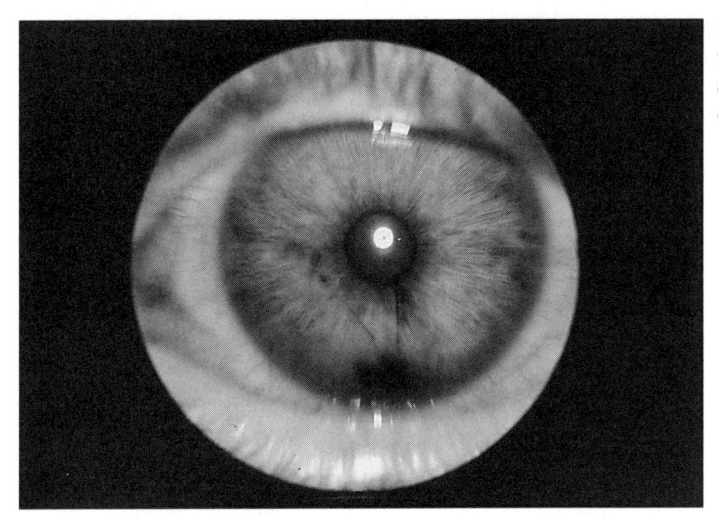

Figure 7-3. Hyphema with iris vessels. (Photograph courtesy of Virginia Mason Medical Center.)

pooling of blood in the anterior chamber, decreased vision, pain, and increased IOP (Figure 7-3). It is important to note that most anterior chamber bleeding comes from the ciliary body. The presence of a hyphema necessitates an urgent status, as the eye may be lacerated or ruptured. Treatment includes restricting movement (bed rest in severe cases), dilating drops, and topical steroids. Usually the body will absorb the hemorrhage on its own, but surgical removal of the blood may be necessary in severe or persistent cases.

Choroid

Blunt trauma may cause choroidal hemorrhages. These may be small and confined to the subretinal layers (appearing as slightly elevated, round, reddish-blue spots with pink edges). This type of choroidal heme usually occurs around the disk or at the equator. They generally clear up after several weeks, but may leave a pigmented area behind. Alternately, the force of the trauma may cause the choroid to bleed into the retinal layers and/or vitreous. It is also possible that the choroid may detach or tear.

Choroidal Prolapse

If the sclera is lacerated, uveal material may exude (prolapse) through the wound. Such a prolapse looks like an oozing of brownish-black fluid on the scleral surface. The pupil may be irregular, often pulled (peaked) up toward the lacerated area. This occurs because the iris is being drawn outward toward the wound. If a patient phones in or presents with these signs, cover the eye at once with a shield. *Do not* apply pressure. Contact the physician at once; this is an emergency situation. If the uveal tissue is exposed to the atmosphere for more than an hour, the chances of developing sympathetic ophthalmia (see next section) are greatly increased.

Sympathetic Ophthalmia

Where there has been a penetrating injury (accidental or surgical) to one eye, the uninjured eye may be at risk for developing sympathetic ophthalmia. This seems to occur more frequently if the choroid or other uveal structures of the injured eye were exposed for an hour or more. It often occurs between 2 to 8 weeks of the original injury, with most cases developing within 12 months. It is believed to be an immunological response, perhaps a sensitization to ocular pigment (which is abundant in the uvea).

The injury may be healing and the eye relatively quiet, but the traumatized eye will be painful and sensitive to light, and the patient will note decreased vision consistent with a low-grade uveitis. The uninjured eye then begins to "sympathize" with its fellow, also developing discomfort (pain, photophobia, and tearing) and blurred vision. The result is a bilateral panuveitis ("pan" means widespread) with all its symptoms and signs. The presence of small yellow-white infiltrates in the retinal pigment epithelium (RPE) is generally the sign that sympathetic ophthalmia is occurring.

Severe vision loss or blindness may result. The more severe the inflammation, the worse the prognosis. In some cases, the signs and symptoms are so subtle that the diagnosis is missed. Treatment involves the use of topical and systemic steroids. Enucleation of the injured eye within 9 to 14 days of the original insult will prevent sympathetic ophthalmia from occurring. However, this is generally recommended only when there is no possibility that the injured eye will recover. Once sympathetic ophthalmia has begun, enucleating the injured eye will not help.

Chapter 8

Emergencies and Injuries of the Vitreous and Retina

Linda Sims, COT

KEY POINTS

- The retina is the light-sensing tissue of the eye.
- Flashes and floaters can be a precursor to an RD or a symptom of a vitreous detachment.
- An RD will usually be accompanied by symptoms of a veil, curtain, or area of darkness in the patient's field of vision.
- Patients with new retinal symptoms need to be seen on an emergent or urgent basis.
- Diabetes, high myopia, and previous eye trauma (including surgery) all may be contributing factors to retinal disease.

Anatomy of the Vitreous and Retina

The vitreous (also called the vitreous humor) is the transparent, gel-like substance that occupies the vitreous cavity. It makes up two-thirds of the volume and three-quarters of the weight of the eye. The vitreous is attached to the retina anteriorly at the ora serrata (the junction of the retina and the ciliary body) and posteriorly at the macula, the large retinal blood vessels, and the margin of the optic nerve.

The retina is the thin, transparent layer of the light-sensing tissue that lines the posterior inside wall of the eye. The retina is made up of many layers of cells and is actually an extension of the brain. It converts light images into electrical impulses that travel via the optic nerve fiber layer and the optic nerve to the brain. The main cell layers include the ganglion cells, the bipolar (connecting) cells, and the rods and cones (the photoreceptor cells) (Figure 8-1).

The posterior layer of the retina is called the pigment epithelium which is attached to the choroid by molecules that act as a sort of "glue," as well as by an osmotic pumping action in the eye. This "pump" is created as fluid within the eye is drawn through the retina toward the wall of the eye. The retina is also firmly attached anteriorly to the ciliary body at the ora serrata and posteriorly at the circumference of the optic nerve.

The retina receives nourishment from blood vessels on its surface and from choroidal vessels underneath its surface. The central retinal artery enters the eye and the central retinal vein exits the eye at the optic disk.

Different areas of the retina include the peripheral retina (which makes up 95% of the retina, contains mainly rod cells, and is responsible for peripheral vision), and the macula (which contains most of the cone cells and is responsible for our fine, colored central vision). The center of the macula is called the fovea (Figure 8-2).

The retina maps images in reverse. Images above the eye are seen with the inferior portion of the retina, while images below the eye are seen with the superior portion of the retina. Likewise, images located temporally are seen with the nasal area of the retina and images located nasally are seen with the temporal area of the retina. This reversal is an important key to locating a retinal problem when the patient is experiencing disturbances in the visual field.

Abnormalities in, or damage to the retina, the optic nerve, or the retinal blood supply can result in vision loss.

Emergencies of the Vitreous

Posterior Vitreous Detachment

Vitreous changes occur as a normal part of aging. The vitreous gel liquifies, condenses, and forms stringy strands. These strands may appear in the vision as small floating circles, spots, or threads. As the vitreous shrinks, it pulls on the retina, causing electrical impulses that the brain perceives as flashes of light. The vitreous may eventually pull free and separate from the posterior retina (posterior vitreous detachment) causing no problems, or it can pull hard enough on the retina to cause a tear, which can lead to a retinal detachment. High myopes and those who have had previous eye surgery, trauma, or inflammation are at higher risk for problems associated with vitreous shrinkage.

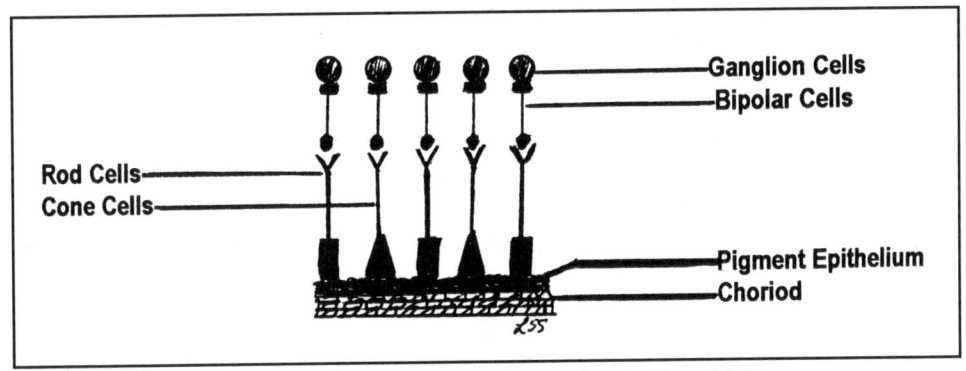

Figure 8-1. Schematic of a retinal cell layer. (Illustration by LS Sims, COT.)

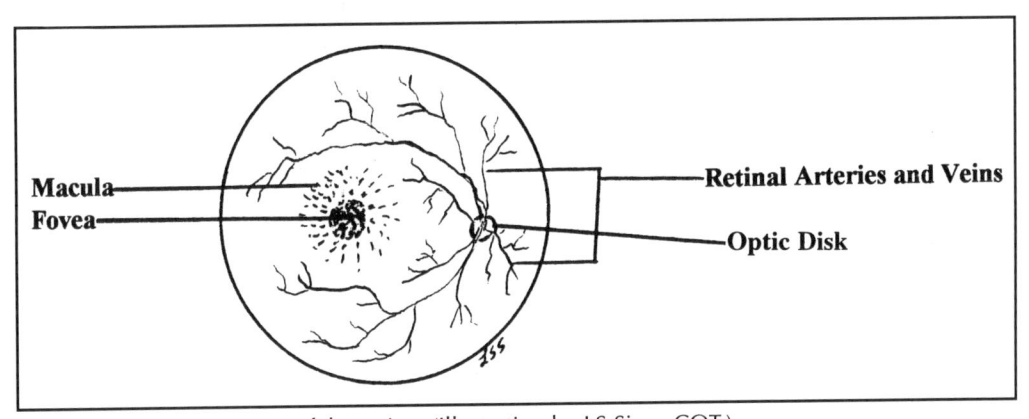

Figure 8-2. Schematic map of the retina. (Illustration by LS Sims, COT.)

Vitreous Hemorrhage

A vitreous hemorrhage occurs when the vitreous shrinks and pulls on the retina, causing a retinal tear in an area which overlies a blood vessel (Figure 8-3). The result is bleeding into the vitreous cavity. The patient may report this as floaters, black dots, swarms of flies, strings, or cobwebs in his or her vision. If there is a great deal of bleeding, vision may become quite dark. Floaters may be accompanied by flashes of light as the vitreous tugs on the retina. When a tear is present, there is the possibility of fluid leaking through the tear, working its way under the retina, lifting it, and causing a detachment. As a general rule, a patient reporting flashes of light accompanied by new floaters and vision changes should be seen on an emergent basis.

Avulsion of the Vitreous Base

Avulsion is a tearing or separation of any part of the body from the whole. Avulsion of the vitreous base can occur as a result of blunt trauma. As the vitreous is torn away from the retina, the patient may notice flashes and floaters, or there may be no noticeable symptoms. Usually no treatment is necessary, but the patient should be warned of signs of an RD.

Figure 8-3. Vitreous hemorrhage. (Photograph courtesy of the Virginia Mason Medical Center.)

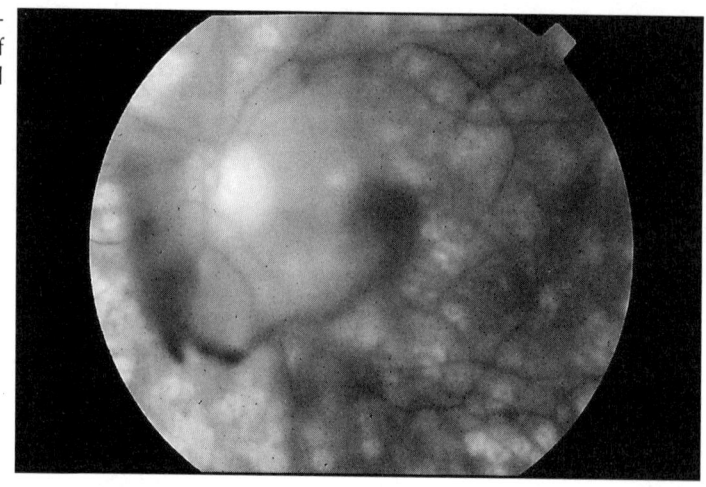

Emergencies of the Retina

Retinal Tears and Detachments

A tear or hole in the retina most often occurs when the vitreous tugs on the retina because of vitreous shrinkage. The vitreous fluid can move through the hole or tear and lift the retina away from the eye wall. If left untreated, the detachment continues until the patient is totally blind in that eye.

The patient will usually (but not always) report symptoms of flashing lights (from the pulling action of the vitreous) and floaters (from the bleeding of broken blood vessels). As the detachment progresses, a shadow, curtain, cloud, or veil may come across a portion of the vision as the photoreceptor layer separates from the nerve fiber layer. A patient reporting such symptoms should be seen on an emergent basis. There is no pain, redness, or discharge associated with an RD alone.

RDs usually begin in the peripheral retina and vision is lost in the corresponding visual field. (For example, a nasally located detachment will appear in the patient's temporal visual field.) If the macula is not affected by the detachment, the central vision may still be 20/20. If the macula detaches, vision drops to 20/400 or worse. If left untreated, irreversible blindness will result. As the retina detaches, it loses contact with its blood supply and dies. Detachments can occur within minutes or take months, but they most commonly form within days. Treatment is surgical. If the macula is "on" (ie, macula is unaffected by the detachment), surgery is done on a more urgent basis, usually within 24 hours. If the detachment is arrested, the macula may be saved. Once the macula is "off" (detached), surgery is considered less urgent and is usually done within days. When the macula is detached, central vision will never be good even if reattachment is successful.

Surgical treatment can include a vitrectomy, scleral buckle, pneumatic retinopexy, cryotherapy, and/or laser treatment (Figure 8-4). A vitrectomy involves removal of the vitreous gel from the eye and replacing it with a saline solution, thereby releasing vitreous traction. A scleral buckle can also be performed, in which a silicone band is placed on top of the sclera to push the outside of the eye wall inward toward the retina. A pneumatic retinopexy is the injection of a gas

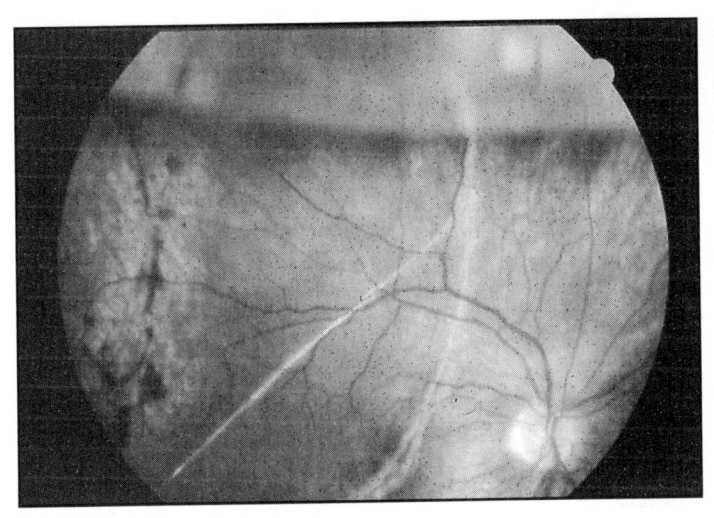

Figure 8-4. RD, s/p laser, and pneumatic retinopexy. (Photograph courtesy of the Virginia Mason Medical Center.)

bubble into the eye to push the retina against the interior eye wall. (In order for the bubble to be effective, the patient must maintain a head position that allows the bubble to float up against the detached area). Cryotherapy is a freezing procedure that creates scar tissue to surround or close a retinal hole or tear. Laser treatments can also be used to create scar tissue via laser burns to surround or close a retinal hole or tear. Commonly, a combination of these treatments are used. For more details about ocular surgery, see Basic Bookshelf title *Overview of Ocular Surgery and Surgical Counseling*.

Macular Holes

A retinal hole that develops in the macular area of the retina is called a macular hole (Figure 8-5). The vitreous that is attached to the macula contracts and pulls up the center of the macula. The patient may notice slight visual disturbances or decreased vision at first. As the vitreous continues to pull, the macula may develop a hole and central vision is lost. A vitrectomy, combined with a pneumatic retinopexy, may improve vision somewhat. A patient with a sudden onset of central vision changes should be seen on an urgent basis.

Retinal Hemorrhage and Edema

Neovascularization, or abnormal new blood vessel growth, may take place in patients with such problems as diabetes or wet macular degeneration. A retinal hemorrhage occurs when these blood vessels leak, causing the retina to become wet and swollen (Figures 8-6 and 8-7). In background diabetic retinopathy (BDR), normal retinal blood vessels develop tiny leaks. In proliferative diabetic retinopathy (PDR), some of the normal blood vessels close, cutting off nutrition to a portion of the retina. The area that is deprived of nutrition will not function properly, and new, abnormal blood vessels will begin to grow. This neovascularization is bad for the eye because the new vessels bleed easily, and scar tissue can form. This entire scenario can result in a total loss of vision.

Retinal hemorrhage and edema can cause blurred vision, while vitreous hemorrhages can cause floaters. If bleeding is profuse, vision may be blocked by what the patient may describe as a swarm of insects in the vision. The patient should be seen on an urgent basis as laser treatment

Figure 8-5. Macular hole. (Photograph courtesy of the Virginia Mason Medical Center.)

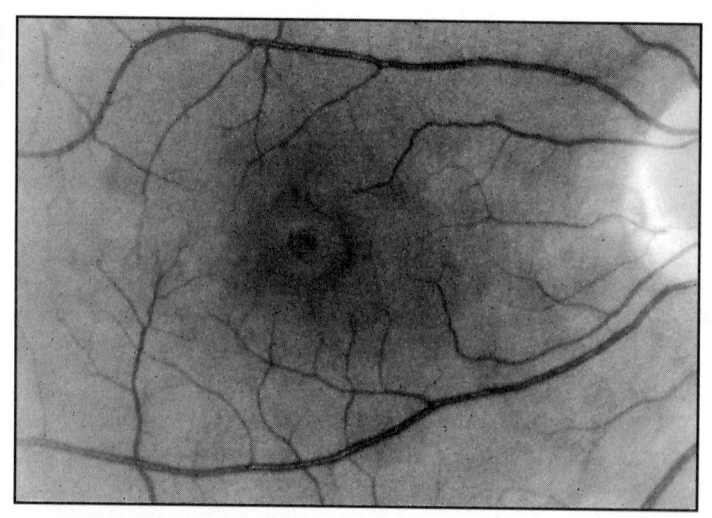

Figure 8-6. Retinal hemorrhage in a leukemia patient. (Photograph courtesy of the Virginia Mason Medical Center.)

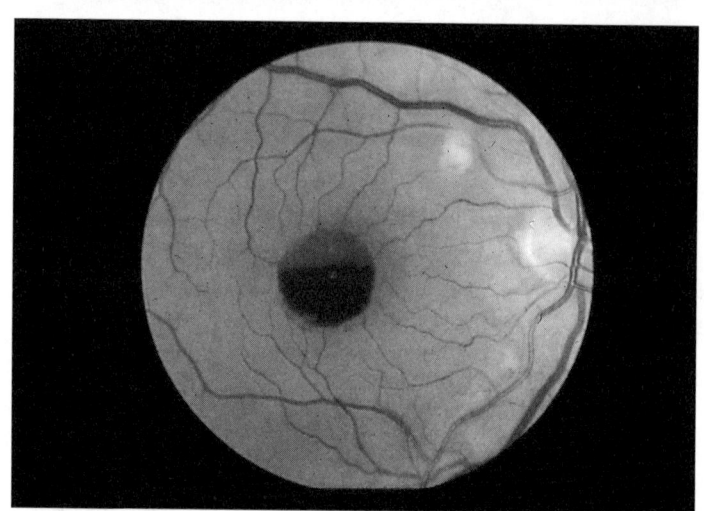

Figure 8-7. Cystoid macular edema. (Photograph courtesy of the Virginia Mason Medical Center.)

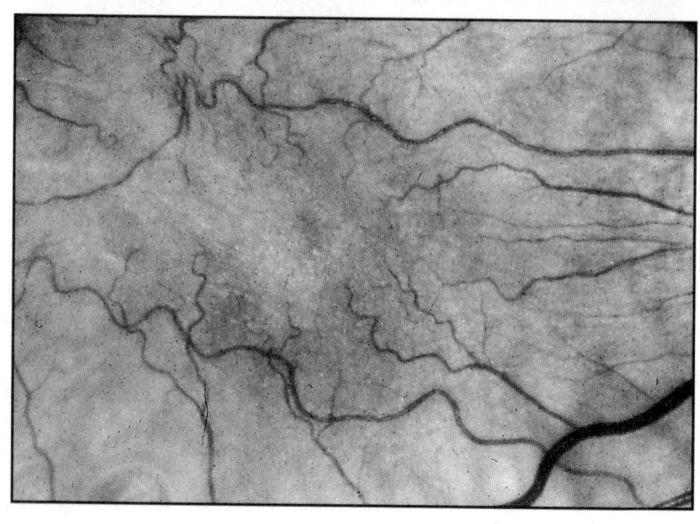

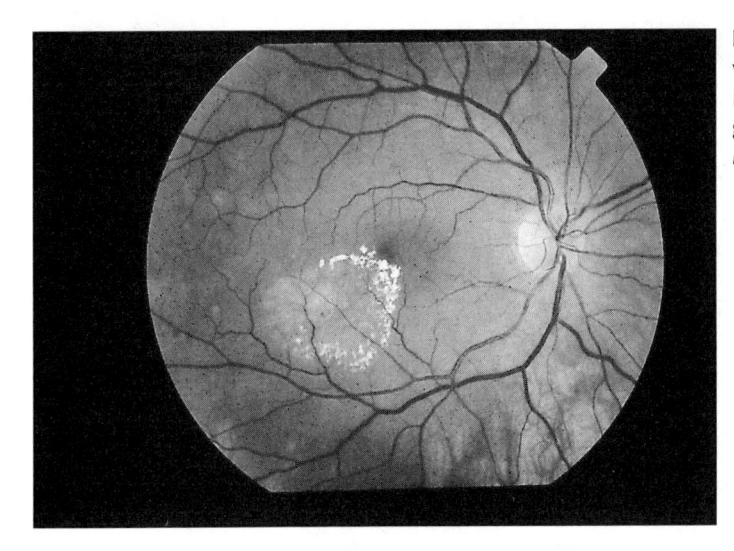

Figure 8-8. Macular edema with ring of exudates, following laser treatment. (Photograph courtesy of the Virginia Mason Medical Center.)

may be used in many cases to seal off the leaking blood vessels. A vitrectomy may become necessary if a vitreous hemorrhage does not clear on its own.

Wet macular degeneration is similar to PDR in that there is neovascularization present. The abnormal blood vessels grow under the retina (lifting it up) and may leak fluid. Since the macula is involved, laser treatment may not be possible because the treatment would damage more of the macula. In some cases, however, laser treatment may be used to stop or retard the neovascularization. Vision will not improve after a laser treatment of this sort; in fact, immediate vision may be worse. However, vision loss from the laser treatment may be less than the eventual vision loss that would occur without any treatment (Figure 8-8). Since macular degeneration is caused by the aging process, laser treatment results may only be temporary. The doctor and patient must weigh the risks and benefits of treatment.

Vascular Occlusions

Vascular occlusions occur as a result of interrupted blood flow to the blood vessels of eye due to blockage.

Central Retinal Artery Occlusions (CRAO)

A CRAO is a true ocular emergency. When the central retinal artery becomes blocked by an embolus (an abnormal particle circulating in the blood), the blood supply is cut off to most layers of the retina, and the tissue dies (Figure 8-9). If the patient is seen within 30 minutes, there is a chance of saving some vision by dilating the retinal arteries enough to allow the blockage to move on into a peripheral arteriole branch (Figure 8-10). This allows some blood flow back into the central retina. Symptoms are a sudden, painless, acute loss of vision in the affected eye. The patient must come in and be treated within 30 minutes. The prognosis without prompt treatment is a permanent and total loss of light perception in the affected eye.

Central Retinal Vein Occlusion (CRVO)

A CRVO can occur in the central retinal vein or in a branch of the retinal vein, and is generally caused by a thrombus (a blood clot that remains attached to its place of origin in a blood ves-

Figure 8-9. CRAO. (Photograph courtesy of Leslie Hargis-Greenshields.)

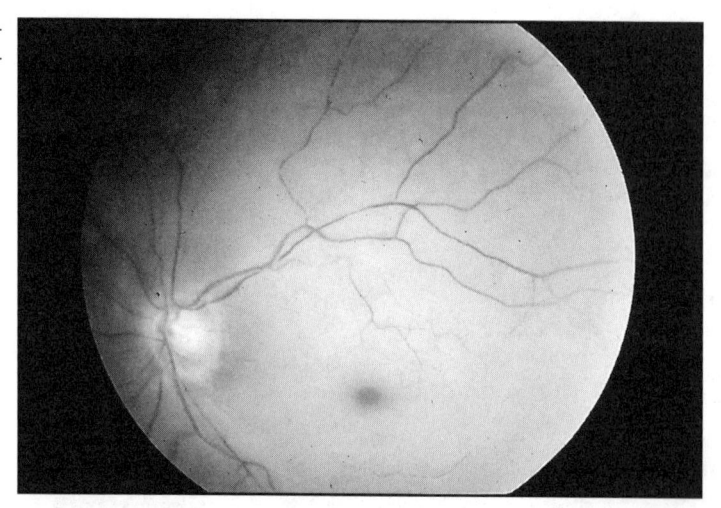

Figure 8-10. Branch retinal artery occlusion (BRAO). (Photograph courtesy of the Virginia Mason Medical Center.)

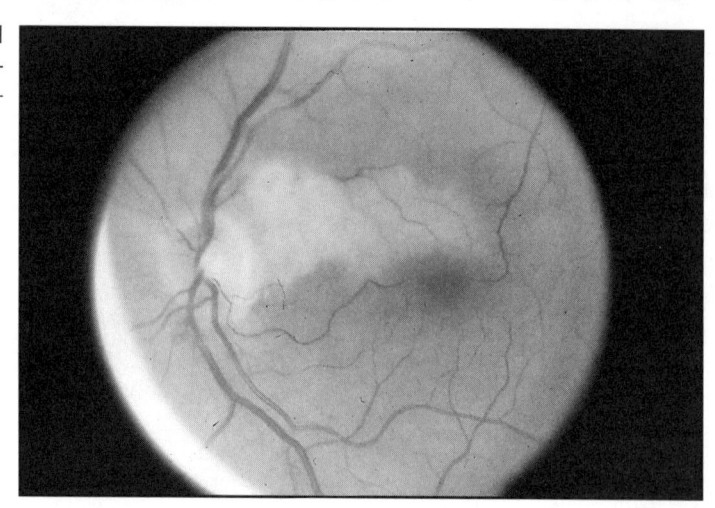

sel). Diabetes, hypertension, glaucoma, cigarette smoking, and age are among factors that increase the risk of CRVOs. Although the condition can be bilateral, most cases are unilateral. Symptoms are often unnoticed at first. There is no pain. With a branch retinal vein occlusion (BRVO) (Figure 8-11), only the vision in the area which the vein passes may be affected. In contrast, in a CRVO (Figure 8-12), central vision will be affected.

On ophthalmoscopic examination, the presence of flame-shaped retinal hemorrhages and cotton-wool spots can be seen along the affected vein, which appears dilated. CRVOs can cause neovascularization on the retina's surface. Such neovascularization can lead to vitreous hemorrhages, edema, RD, and neovascular glaucoma. A fluorescein angiogram is usually taken to determine the extent of blood flow interruption, and a panretinal laser photocoagulation may be performed to curb the neovascularization. Prognosis for a CRVO is poor, with good visual recovery unlikely. A person noticing a sudden change in their central or peripheral vision should be seen on an urgent basis.

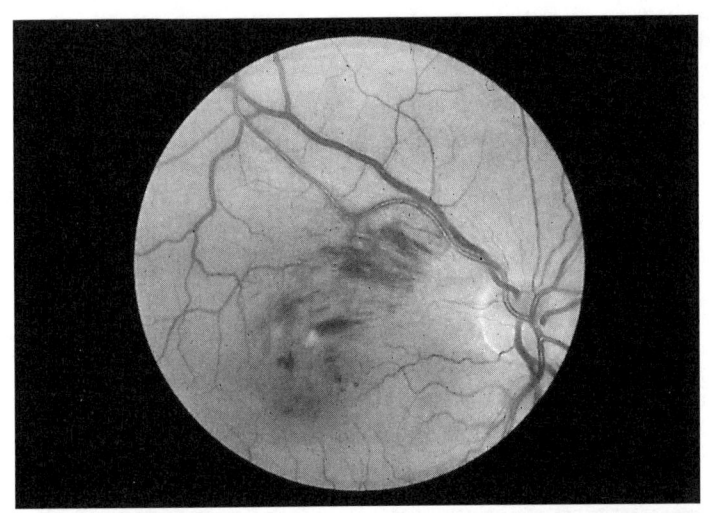

Figure 8-11. BRVO. (Photograph courtesy of the Virginia Mason Medical Center.)

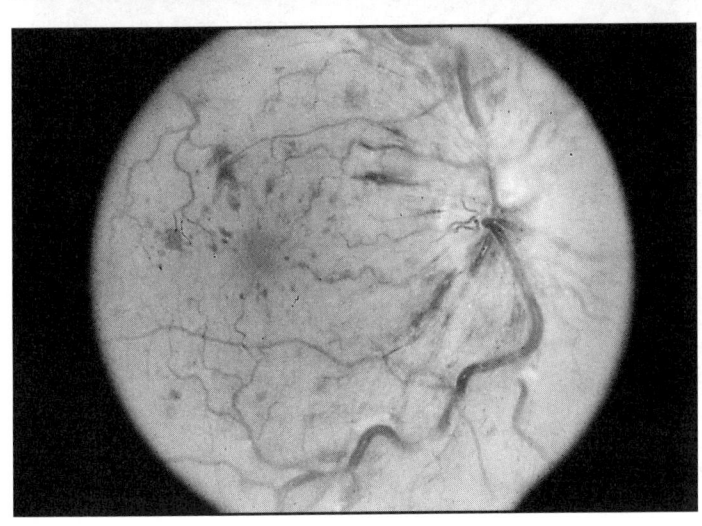

Figure 8-12. CRVO. (Photograph courtesy of the Virginia Mason Medical Center.)

Posterior Segment Trauma

Trauma to the posterior segment of the eye can be classified into blunt trauma, penetrating or perforating injuries (Figure 8-13), intraocular FBs (Figure 8-14), or trauma due to distant injury. A patient phoning about any eye injury should be seen on an urgent basis. A complete history needs to be obtained when the trauma patient is first examined. The history should include the manner and time of injury, if it was work related, what emergency care was carried out prior to arrival, the status of the eye before the injury, and the time when the patient last ate or drank (should surgery be necessary). If the patient is able, check the visual acuity. Do not put any pressure on an injured eye.

Blunt Trauma

Blunt trauma occurs in injuries where an object contacts but does not penetrate the eye. The damage is caused by the transmission of force from the moving object to the eye tissue. Damage can be minor and transient, or may result in a permanent loss of vision.

Figure 8-13. Perforated globe. (Printed with permission from Herrin M. *Ophthalmic Examination and Basic Skills.* Thorofare, NJ: SLACK Incorporated; 1990.)

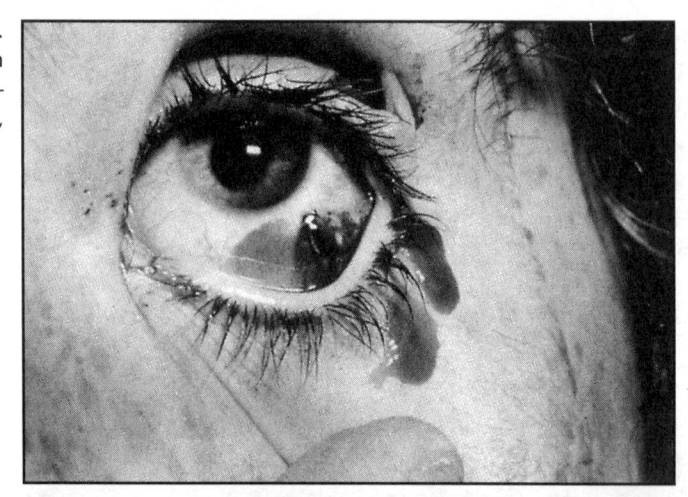

Figure 8-14. Intraocular glass FB. (Photograph courtesy of TD Lindquist, MD, PhD.)

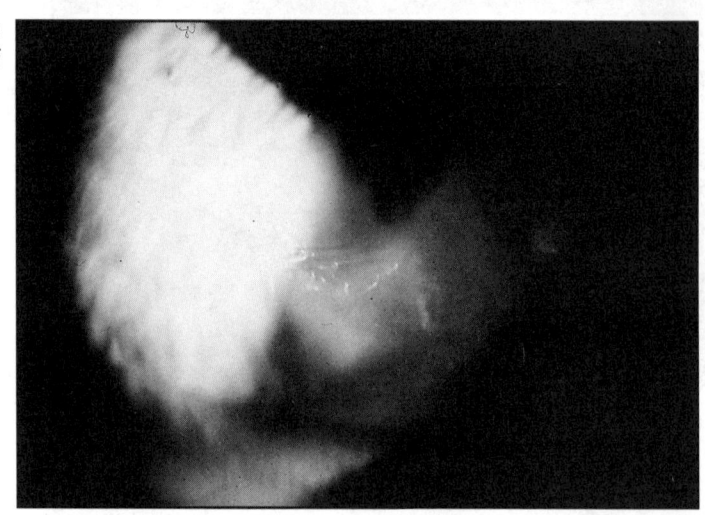

Vitreous Hemorrhage

Vitreous hemorrhage can result from blood vessel damage, retinal tears, or scleral rupture. If the hemorrhage is so dense that the retina cannot be seen on exam, an ultrasound test may be used to detect the damaged area. The hemorrhage will generally clear with time, but the prognosis depends on the area and extent of injury.

Traumatic Detachment

Compression expands the globe, creating traction in the vitreous base. This traction is transmitted to the peripheral retina, which is normally firmly attached to the vitreous. As the retina is compressed it pulls on the vitreous, creating a tear or detachment. Such a detachment can occur from one week to two years after the original injury.

Commotio Retinae (Berlin's Edema)

Commotio retinae refers to extensive, patchy swelling of the retina that can form within minutes to hours after blunt trauma to the anterior segment. The retinal area opposite the site of impact is involved. White opacified patches with ill-defined borders are seen on the retina. (This condition can be differentiated from a CRAO because there is normal blood flow through the inner retinal vessels). Visual acuity usually returns slowly over several weeks.

Macular Edema

Macular edema and macular hole formation can result from a blunt traumatic injury. The fovea is very thin, and blunt trauma can cause contusion necrosis (death of the cells in a localized area), subfoveal hemorrhage, and/or vitreous traction. Any time the macula is involved, central vision will be affected.

Choroidal Rupture

A choroidal rupture is a break in the pigmented blood vessels of the choroid layer that lies under the retina. Central vision will be involved if the macula is affected. Subretinal neovascularization can later form in areas of choroidal rupture, with associated hemorrhage and scarring.

Optic Nerve Injuries

Optic nerve injuries can occur from an interruption of blood flow, compression (from swelling and/or fractured orbital bones after a blunt trauma), laceration (by fractured orbital bones or intraorbital FB), or concussion (from frontal or temporal head injuries).

Avulsion of the optic nerve can occur under several circumstances, such as extreme turning and forward dislocation of the globe, a penetrating injury that causes a backward pull on the optic nerve, or sudden increase in IOP.

Symptoms of an optic nerve injury can include decreased vision, pain (associated with the traumatic injury), afferent pupillary defect, relatively poor color vision, and/or a visual field defect.

Treatment can consist of antibiotic and steroid medications and surgical intervention. Prognosis is dependent on the type and extent of injury. However, once the optic nerve is severed, vision is irretrievable.

Papilledema is a swelling of the optic disk associated with elevated intracranial pressure (pressure within the skull). There may be a transient vision loss (lasting seconds), and/or diplopia, but often vision is normal except for an enlarged physiological blind spot. Other symptoms can include headaches and nausea. Treatment and prognosis is dependent on the underlying cause of the intracranial pressure.

Rupture of the Globe

Blunt trauma, if severe, can cause the globe to rupture. The two most common sites of rupture are at the limbus and under the insertions of the rectus muscles. These points are the weakest points of the sclera. Signs of rupture include a decrease in ocular movement, conjunctival chemosis and hemorrhage. Normal vision may not be salvageable because the force required to rupture the globe is so intense that injury to the eye is usually extensive. The presence of an intraocular FB must be ruled out anytime a globe is ruptured.

Penetrating and Perforating Injuries

A penetrating injury occurs when a sharp object cuts or tears the eye wall. A perforating injury has both an entrance and exit wound, and occurs when a sharp object passes through the eye. These injuries can result from an assault, a motor vehicle accident, an industrial accident, any type of projectile (such as a BB pellet or piece of metal), or sharp objects such as a needle or knife. Signs and symptoms include decreased vision, decreased IOP, a change in the anterior chamber depth, a displaced or irregularly shaped pupil, a visible wound to the cornea or sclera, prolapse of ocular tissues, and/or chemosis of the conjunctiva. Penetration of the globe should always be suspected when even small lid lacerations are present. If penetration to the globe is suspected, do not instill drops or apply pressure. Cover with an eye shield and notify the physician at once.

Intraocular Foreign Bodies

Each case of an intraocular FB injury is unique. The direct trauma to the orbital structures may be associated with hemorrhage, edema, infection and post-traumatic scarring. Complications can range from decreased vision, to loss of vision, to loss of an eye. The potential for damage beyond the orbit is always a concern because of the eye's proximity to the brain and the paranasal sinuses. Treatment includes surgical removal of the FB and systemic antibiotics. Any suspicion of an intraocular FB should be treated on an emergent basis.

Metallic Foreign Bodies

Siderosis bulbi is a pathological condition of iron toxicity caused by a retained iron FB. The metal causes a degenerative loss of vision as iron saturates the entire retina over a span of 2 months to 2 years. Iron toxicity can also affect the trabecular meshwork, leading to glaucoma. The iris may also change color. If the FB is removed at an early stage, toxicity may be prevented.

Chalcosis is a pathological condition of copper deposition in eye tissues caused by an FB with a copper content of 70% or more, and can lead to cataracts or glaucoma. A copper content of 90% or more can cause a massive purulent inflammation, while a copper content of less than 70% will rarely cause intraocular problems.

Metals such as gold, silver, platinum, zinc, and aluminum are chemically inert and cause no damage other than disruption of tissues due to penetration.

Non-Metallic Foreign Bodies

Organic FBs, such as twigs or tree branches, can lead to fungal or bacterial infections and endophthalmitis. Other non-metallic FBs include glass and plastic, which cause no damage other than that occurring with the penetrating injury (unless contaminated by organic matter).

Posterior Eye Injury Due to Distant Injury

Retinal damage may result from injuries not directly involving the eye, such as head, neck, and chest injuries.

Purtscher's Retinopathy

Purtscher's retinopathy may occur in one or both eyes following a head or chest compression injury. It is thought to be caused by a rapid rise in the pressure of the cerebrospinal fluid. This pressure is transmitted to the central vein in the optic nerve. On retinal exam, white patchy exudates can be seen close to the retinal veins and small hemorrhages are visible all around the posterior pole. These findings appear within the first two days after injury. Visual acuity may or may not be impaired, depending on the degree of macular involvement. Prognosis is also dependent on macular involvement. No treatment is available.

Shaken Baby Syndrome

Shaken baby syndrome is a form of child abuse that includes severe shaking of an infant, causing a whiplash-type of injury. General signs include bradycardia (slow heart beat), apnea (transient suspension of respiration), hypothermia, irritability, lethargy, and skin bruises. Retinal signs include retinal hemorrhages and cotton wool spots, principally involving the macular area. The progression of the hemorrhages can help date the incident. The physician should report suspected cases of child abuse to the appropriate authorities.

Endophthalmitis

Endophthalmitis is an infection of the vitreous and surrounding tissues, usually caused by bacteria. It can occur postoperatively, post-traumatically (especially secondary to a penetrating injury or intraocular FB), or endogenously (from within the body through systemic circulation). Endophthalmitis is more frequent in the elderly and in postoperative glaucoma patients who have a filtering bleb. Signs and symptoms include a sudden onset of reduced vision, pain, redness, corneal haze, and sometimes a hypopyon.

The infection can destroy the eye within days. If treatment is delayed by even 24 hours, good visual recovery will be less likely. If endophthalmitis is suspected, the patient should be seen on an emergent basis. Treatment includes massive doses of antibiotics administered topically, periocularly, intraocularly, and systemically.

Chapter 9

The Red Eye

OptT
OphA
CL

Linda Sims, COT

KEY POINTS

- The red eye is a pathological condition in which the blood vessels of the conjunctiva or ciliary body become dilated. This can signify a serious vision-threatening condition or a superficial transient irritation.
- Tissues of the lids, lacrimal system, and orbit may also become red and inflamed due to pathological conditions.
- The most common causes of the red eye are irritation and infection. Other causes include allergic reaction, disease, and trauma.
- Eye redness with itching usually indicates an allergic reaction.
- Eye redness with an acute onset of a poking or sticking pain suggests the presence of an FB or corneal abrasion.
- Eye redness with deep internal pain can signify glaucoma, uveitis, or scleritis.
- Eye redness with burning, irritation, and/or a gritty feeling suggests a superficial condition of the lids, conjunctiva, or cornea.

Introduction

When we think of the "red eye," we almost immediately think of angle-closure glaucoma, iritis, and conjunctivitis. The first is emergent, the second urgent, and the third rarely serious. However, there are other emergent and urgent causes of red eye besides angle-closure and iritis. Cellulitis, scleritis, endophthalmitis, and injury are examples. Yet these may vie for same-day appointments with non-emergent cases such as subconjunctival hemorrhages, dry eye, and styes, all of which may be uncomfortable or alarming and therefore seem urgent to the patient.

A list of possible causes of a condition is called a "differential diagnosis." Once we have the patient's chief complaint, we must mentally scroll through the potential causative factors to be able to ask key questions that will help narrow down that list enough to determine when the patient needs to be seen. This is especially true when the patient has phoned in with the problem and we don't have the advantage of visual inspection. In order to help in determining a differential diagnosis of red eye, this chapter will also briefly mention non-emergent causes. Because we want this chapter to stand alone, some material covered in previous chapters is again mentioned here.

In general, patients with a painful red eye and vision decrease should be seen on an urgent basis (within 24 to 48 hours). Also, some eye infections and diseases can do serious damage to the eye in a relatively short period of time if left untreated, and should be seen as urgent. Monocular patients relating even questionably serious symptoms should be seen on an urgent basis. When triaging a red eye, do not be afraid to err on the side of caution, and do not hesitate to ask your physician's advice.

Orbit, Lids, and Lacrimal System

The orbit, lids, and lacrimal system (collectively known as the ocular adnexa) are the structures surrounding the eyeball. The tissues of these structures can be affected by irritation, infection, or physiological abnormalities that can lead to itching, pain, and redness. While most diseases and conditions of the ocular adnexa are non-emergent, there are a few that require prompt attention.

Orbital and Preseptal Cellulitis

Cellulitis, an infection or inflammation of tissue, can affect the lids or the orbit.

Orbital Cellulitis

Orbital cellulitis is a potentially life-threatening condition. It produces swollen, red lids and conjunctiva, proptosis (bulging eyes), impaired ocular motility with pain on eye movement, double vision, fever, and headache. If the optic nerve is involved there will also be decreased vision.

Orbital cellulitis is often a secondary infection that begins in the sinuses or other regions of the body and is most commonly caused by the Staphylococcus aureus organism (although other bacteria, viruses, or fungi may be responsible). It should be treated as an emergent condition due to the danger of the infection spreading to the nearby venous sinus of the brain. Treatment includes hospitalization and intravenous antibiotics, later changing to oral antibiotics as the condition improves. An ointment such as erythromycin may also be prescribed if corneal exposure is occurring secondary to proptosis. (See Chapter 3.)

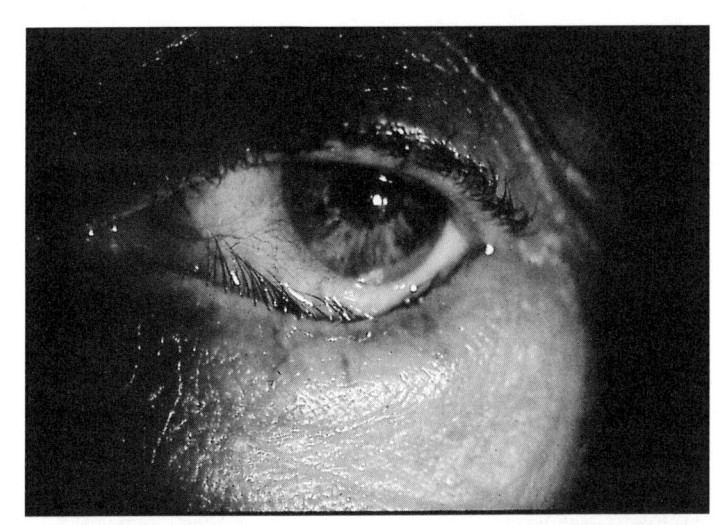

Figure 9-1. Entropion. (Photograph courtesy of EL Hargis, MD.)

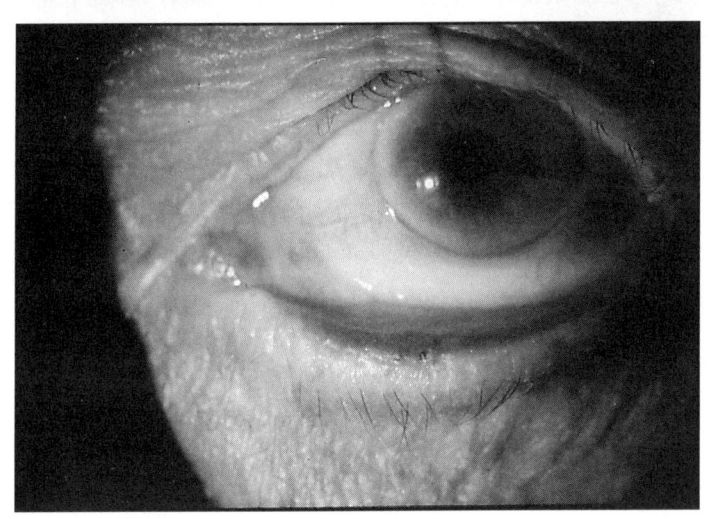

Figure 9-2. Ectropion. (Photograph courtesy of EL Hargis, MD.)

Preseptal Cellulitis

Preseptal cellulitis is characterized by swelling and infection of the lid tissue in front of the orbital septum, causing the skin and lids to be tender and red. However, the patient's vision, pupils, and ocular motility will not be affected. The most common causes of preseptal cellulitis are the Staphylococcus aureus and streptococci organisms. Treatment consists of oral and/or intravenous antibiotics, lid ointment, and warm compresses (see also Chapter 2).

Physical Abnormalities of the Ocular Adnexa

Entropion (an inward turning of the eyelid that can cause the lashes to rub the eye) (Figure 9-1), and ectropion (an outward turning of the eyelid that can cause exposure of the anterior cornea and conjunctiva) (Figure 9-2) are physical abnormalities that may bring on discomfort, tearing, and redness. Treatment is usually surgical correction.

Trichiasis (in which the eyelid is in a normal position but the lashes point inward, rubbing the eye) can cause pain, redness, and corneal damage. Temporary treatment involves simple epilation (plucking) of the offending lashes. A more permanent treatment is electrolysis (a low-level electrical charge applied to the lash root), or cryosurgery (a freezing of the general area of the lash).

The Conjunctiva

The conjunctiva is a thin, transparent membrane that lines the inner surface of the eyelids, continues over the anterior surface of the sclera, and attaches to the cornea at the limbus.

Conjunctivitis

Conjunctivitis, commonly referred to as "pink eye," is an inflammation of the conjunctiva that is characterized by discharge, swelling, grittiness, itching, and burning. While not actually emergent, conjunctivitis is important in any discussion of red eye because of its prominent place in differential diagnosis. Conjunctivitis may be caused by infectious organisms that can be bacterial or viral in nature, or by an allergic reaction to pollen (atopic), eye medications (contact), or seasonal conditions (vernal). The type of discharge present can also help differentiate the cause. A watery discharge is characteristic of viral conjunctivitis. A mucopurulent, or thick mucus and pus-containing, discharge is associated with bacterial conjunctivitis. A watery discharge with white, stringy mucus signifies allergic conjunctivitis.

Bacterial Conjunctivitis

While bacterial and viral conjunctivitis are both contagious and may cause discomfort, most cases are not considered an ocular emergency. One exception is the gonococcal form of bacterial conjunctivitis, a severe infection that can lead to corneal ulceration and blindness if treatment is delayed (Figure 9-3). Gonococcal conjunctivitis is characterized by large amounts of mucopurulent discharge and progresses with symptoms of lid swelling, aching pain, and tenderness. Treatment includes systemic antibiotics, topical antimicrobial medications, and cycloplegics (if the cornea is involved).

More commonly, bacterial conjunctivitis is caused by the Staphylococcus aureus organism (Figure 9-4). This infection is characterized by a lesser degree of mucopurulent discharge, redness, and discomfort. Staph conjunctivitis tends to resolve spontaneously within 2 weeks without treatment, but topical medications may be used to speed the recovery and increase patient comfort.

Viral Conjunctivitis

Viral organisms are the most common cause of all conjunctival infections. Viral conjunctivitis is usually caused by the adenovirus and is characterized by a watery discharge, redness, and discomfort (Figure 9-5). There is no effective treatment to speed resolution, which usually occurs within 1 to 3 weeks, but drops may be prescribed to lessen symptoms.

Other Types of Conjunctivitis

Allergic conjunctivitis is characterized by itching and burning, and a watery discharge with white stringy mucus (Figure 9-6). Treatment is directed toward alleviating symptoms with topical antihistamines or artificial tears.

Neonatal conjunctivitis occurs in a newborn as a result of exposure to various bacteria or viruses in the birth canal. Silver nitrate drops are routinely used to prevent eye infections in newborns. The silver nitrate may itself produce contact conjunctivitis, but this clears rapidly.

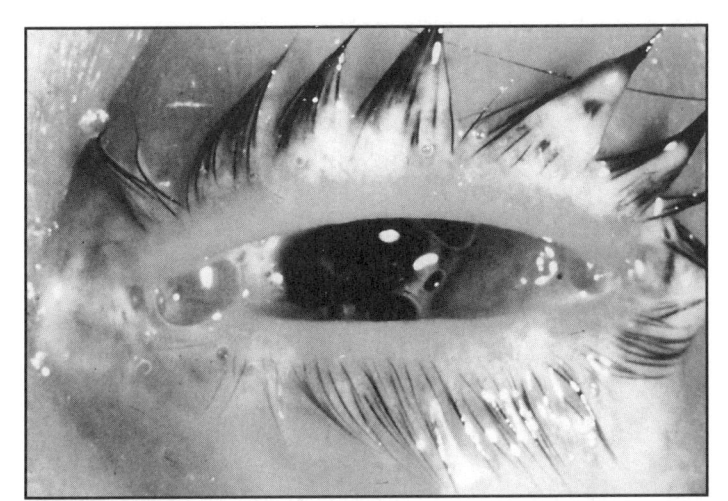

Figure 9-3. Mucopurulent conjunctivitis. (Photograph courtesy of TD Lindquist, MD, PhD.)

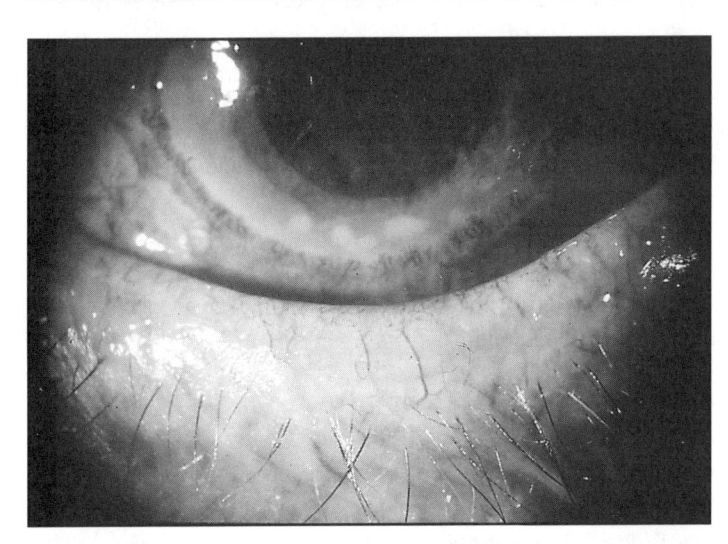

Figure 9-4. Staph marginal disease. (Photograph courtesy of TD Lindquist, MD, PhD.)

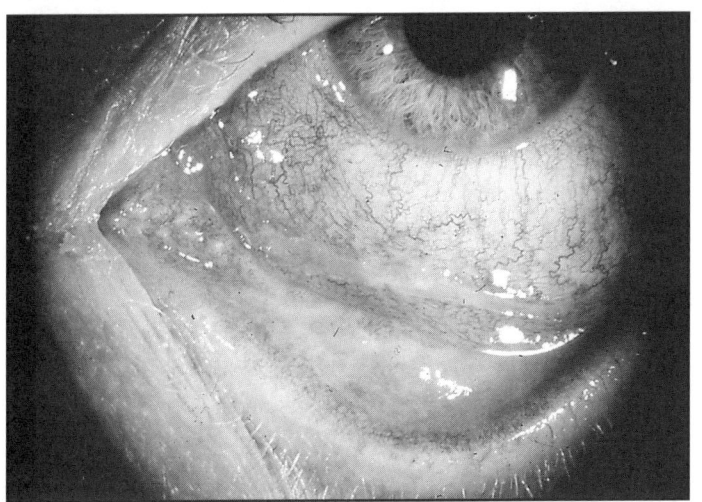

Figure 9-5. Viral conjunctivitis. (Photograph courtesy of TD Lindquist, MD, PhD.)

Figure 9-6. Allergic conjunctivitis. (Photograph courtesy of TD Lindquist, MD, PhD.)

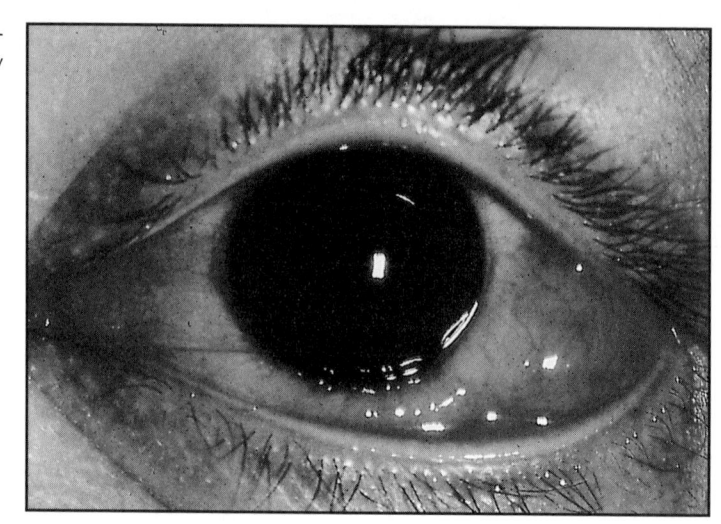

Keratoconjunctivitis Sicca

Keratoconjunctivitis sicca (dry eye) is caused by decreased tear production or a decrease in oil secretion by the meibomian glands, and is common with aging (Figures 9-7 and 9-8). Dry eye may be associated with systemic diseases such as rheumatoid arthritis and Stevens-Johnson syndrome, as well as the use of medications such as diuretics, antihistamines, and antibiotics. Symptoms include an FB sensation, irritation, and redness. Treatment includes use of artificial tears in eyedrop or ointment form. In more severe cases, occlusion of the lacrimal drainage ducts may be accomplished by means of punctal cautery or punctal plugs.

Subconjunctival Hemorrhages

A subconjunctival hemorrhage is a pooling of blood from a broken blood vessel under the clear conjunctival surface (Figure 9-9). The redness is accentuated by the whiteness of sclera. There is no pain or change in vision. While the patient may find the hemorrhage alarming, it is merely like a bruise underneath the skin. The body will reabsorb the blood within 1 to 3 weeks. Subconjunctival hemorrhages may be related to coughing, sneezing, vomiting, lifting or straining, or bleeding disorders (rare). Most commonly no cause can be established. Topical vasoconstrictors are of little, if any, benefit. No treatment is needed, merely reassurance.

Pinguecula and Pterygium

Pinguecula and pterygium are both pathological tissue changes caused by exposure to sun, wind, and dust, and appear as a yellowish or white mass. A pinguecula is a wedge-shaped thickening of the conjunctiva (Figure 9-10). If it extends onto the cornea it is called a pterygium (Figure 9-11). A pterygium can cause loss of vision if it grows across the visual axis of the cornea. Irritants such as smoke and fumes tend to cause a pinguecula or pterygium to become red and inflamed, accentuating its appearance. Treatment includes use of artificial tears for comfort, vasoconstrictors to lessen redness, or surgical removal.

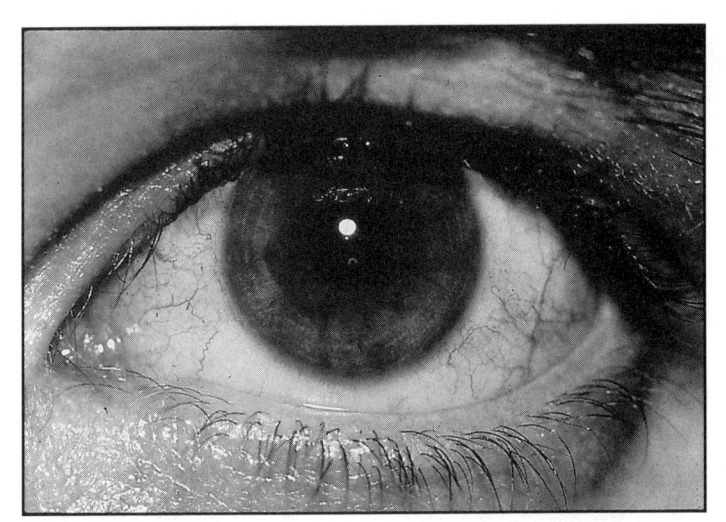

Figure 9-7. Early dry eye. (Photograph courtesy of TD Lindquist, MD, PhD.)

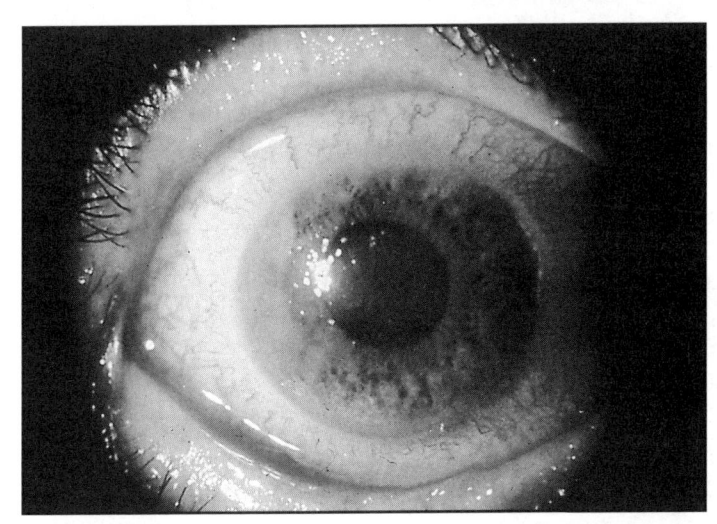

Figure 9-8. Dry eye. (Photograph courtesy of TD Lindquist, MD, PhD.)

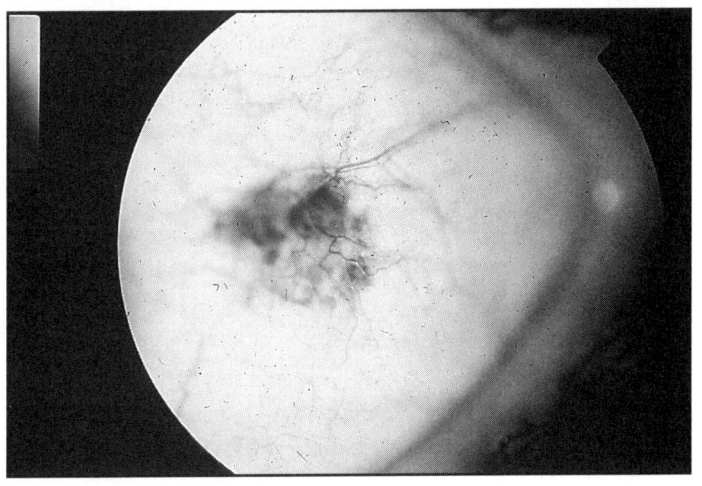

Figure 9-9. Subconjunctival hemorrhage. (Photograph courtesy of LS Sims, COT.)

Figure 9-10. Pinguecula. (Photograph courtesy of EL Hargis, MD.)

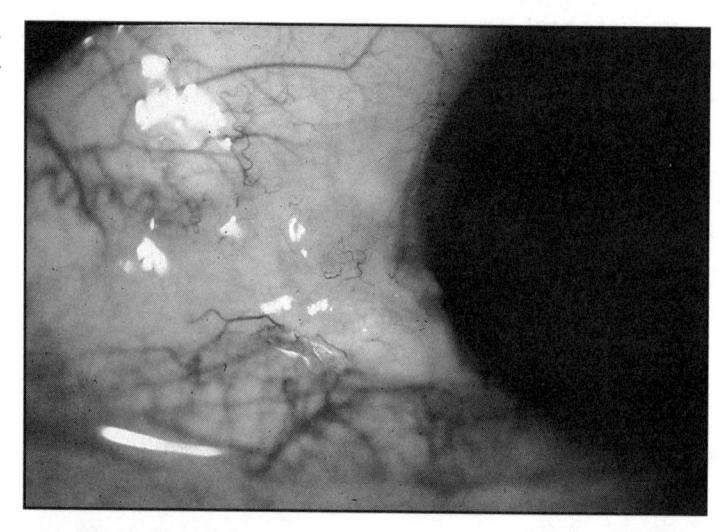

Figure 9-11. Pteryguim. (Photograph courtesy of TD Lindquist, MD, PhD.)

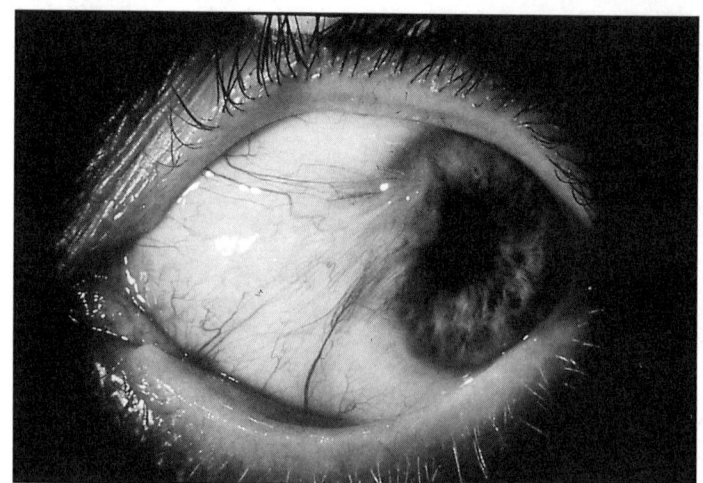

The Sclera

The sclera is the white protective covering that encompasses the globe from the cornea to the optic nerve. Its function is to provide a firm, protective coat for the intraocular contents. The sclera consists of avascular collagen and elastic tissue that allows for variations in IOP, while still providing enough support to prevent distortion of the ocular contents.

Scleritis

Scleritis is a destructive disease that can lead to severe pain, perforation of the globe, vision loss, and/or loss of the eye (Figure 9-12). Early diagnosis and treatment are essential. Symptoms of scleritis include pain, redness, photophobia, and tearing. The normally white sclera may have a bluish hue when observed in natural light. Pain from scleritis will often radiate up into the forehead, brow, or jaw area and be so severe that it wakes the patient at night. Recurrent episodes are common. Scleral disease can be related to disease in other parts of the body. General health questions should be asked regarding cardiovascular, respiratory, autoimmune, and skin diseases.

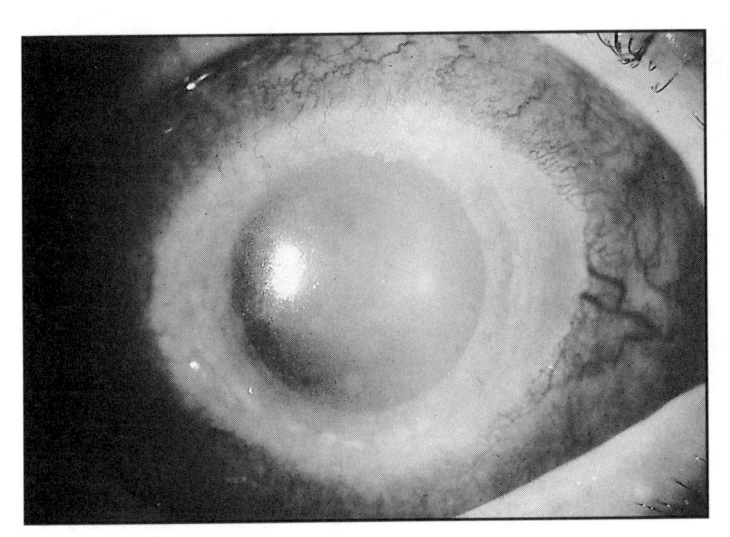

Figure 9-12. Scleritis. (Photograph courtesy of TD Lindquist, MD, PhD.)

Associated anterior chamber inflammation, if present, may lead to secondary glaucoma, corneal endothelial damage, cataract, or posterior synechiae. Scleritis can lead to scleral and corneal thinning, which can lead to perforations. Such perforations may create a portal of entry for a secondary infection. If the thinning is in the posterior sclera area, RDs or optic nerve changes may occur. Since the posterior sclera cannot be directly visualized, the diagnosis is more difficult to make.

Treatment includes non-steroidal anti-inflammatory drugs (such as ibuprofen), systemic steroids, and sometimes the use of steroid drops (for patient comfort). Surgery is rarely needed.

Episcleritis

The episclera is the highly elastic vascular connective tissue that lies between the sclera and the conjunctiva. Conditions affecting only the episclera are usually acute but transient, and of little concern. However, the tissues of the episclera will also show signs of disease when the sclera itself is affected. Therefore it is important for the ophthalmologist to distinguish which scleral tissues are involved. The differential diagnosis may be aided by use of topical phenylephrine. If the condition is episcleritis (Figure 9-13), the inflamed episcleral vessels will blanch shortly after the instillation of phenylephrine. If it is scleritis, inflamed scleral vessels will not blanch with phenyephrine instillation.

Treatment of episcleritis includes artificial tears or a topical vasoconstrictor for mild cases, topical steroids for moderate to severe cases. An NSAID may be prescribed in rare cases.

The Cornea

The cornea is the clear, highly sensitive, avascular "window" at the front of the eye that covers the anterior chamber, iris, and pupil. The majority of the eye's refractive power comes from the cornea. It also provides a tough physical barrier that shields the inside of the eye from bacteria, dust, and other harmful matter.

The cornea is thickest at the edges and thinnest at the center. It is divided into five layers: the epithelium, Bowman's membrane, the stroma, Descemet's membrane, and the endothelium. The

Figure 9-13. Episcleritis. (Photograph courtesy of TD Lindquist, MD, PhD.)

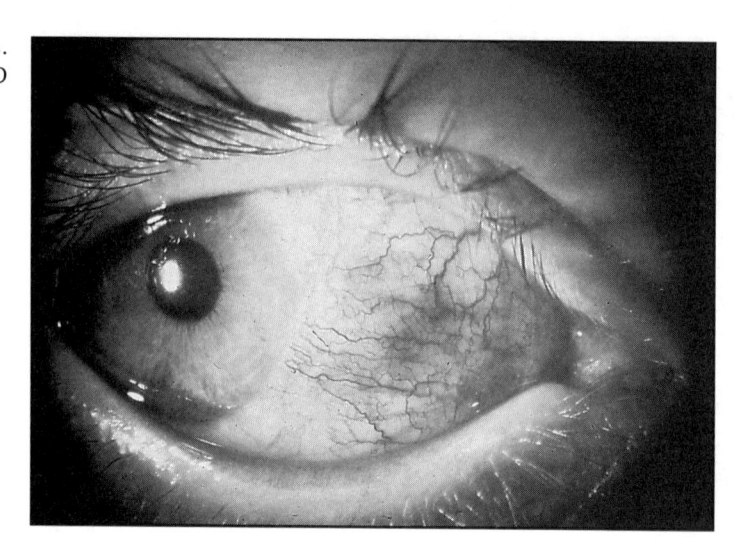

epithelium, the outermost layer, is the part of the cornea most often injured by small foreign bodies or superficial abrasions. The epithelium regenerates quickly and heals without scarring. Injuries to the deepest layers of the cornea usually lead to greater pain, blurred vision, tearing, redness, and extreme photophobia, and can result in corneal opacification and decreased visual acuity. Because of the cornea's vital role in vision, its disorders are generally at least urgent in nature.

Corneal Abrasion

Corneal abrasions occur if the epithelial layer is scratched or scraped (Figure 9-14). This can result from contact lens wear, trauma, or dry eyes. Symptoms include redness, tearing, pain, FB sensation, photophobia, and blurred vision. Abrasions may be treated with topical antibiotics to prevent infection, cycloplegics for comfort, and pressure patching. They usually heal quickly, within 24 to 48 hours.

Recurrent Corneal Erosions

Recurrent corneal erosions (or recurrent erosion syndrome) may occur after a corneal scratch or scrape has healed (Figure 9-15). It can also be associated with dry eye, infections, previous chemical injury, or previous eye surgery. These recurrent erosions result when the epithelium fails to adhere to Bowman's membrane. The patient may awaken with an FB sensation due to the lids being opened or rubbed, which abrades the epithelial layer. Symptoms include pain, photophobia, and tearing. Treatment can include a cycloplegic drop, an antibiotic ointment, and/or a pressure patch for 24 to 48 hours (for acute cases). After the epithelium is healed, artificial tear drops and ointments are prescribed. In cases where the epithelium is loose and not healing, debridement (removal of the affected tissue to aid in healing) may be performed. If the erosion is not responsive to the above treatments, a bandage soft contact lens may be prescribed for several months.

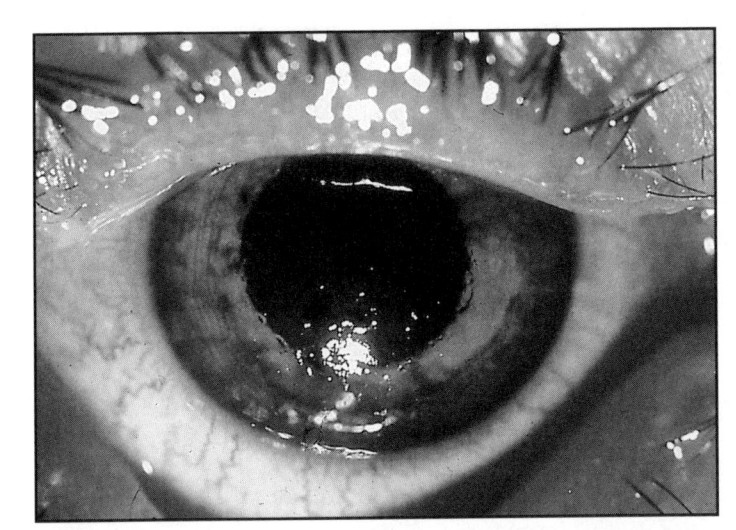

Figure 9-14. Corneal abrasion. (Photograph courtesy of TD Lindquist, MD, PhD.)

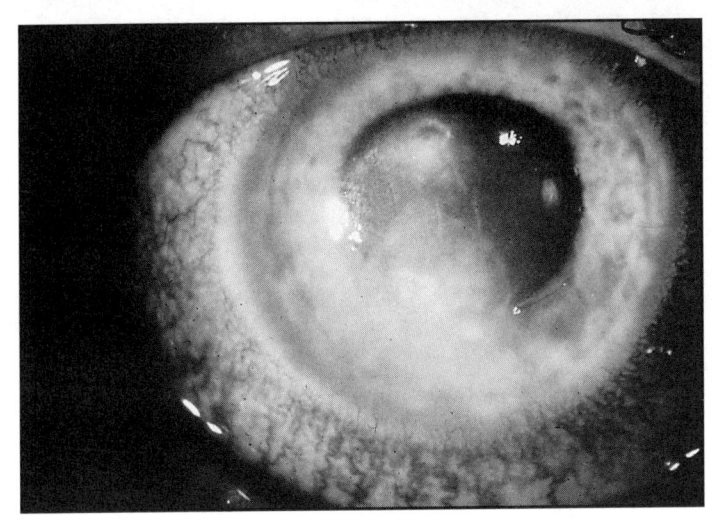

Figure 9-15. Recurrent erosion. (Photograph courtesy of TD Lindquist, MD, PhD.)

Keratitis and Corneal Ulcers

Keratitis is a corneal inflammation characterized by a loss of corneal transparency and accompanied by cellular infiltration (Figure 9-16). It is usually caused by viral or bacterial organisms (discussed next), chemical or physical injury, or high levels of ultraviolet light exposure.

Corneal ulcers occur when there is an area of tissue loss that usually penetrates deeper than the epithelial layer, and is generally accompanied by corneal inflammation and anterior chamber cells (Figure 9-17). Causes can be from viral, bacterial, or fungal organisms, or due to trauma.

Infectious Corneal Keratitis and Ulcers

Ocular herpes is the most common form of viral keratitis. While ocular herpes can result from the sexually transmitted herpes simplex type II virus, it usually caused by the herpes simplex type I virus, the same virus responsible for cold sores. Ocular herpes produces a somewhat painful ulcer on the corneal epithelium with a characteristically dendritic (branch-like) shape

Figure 9-16. Keratitis. (Photograph courtesy of TD Lindquist, MD, PhD.)

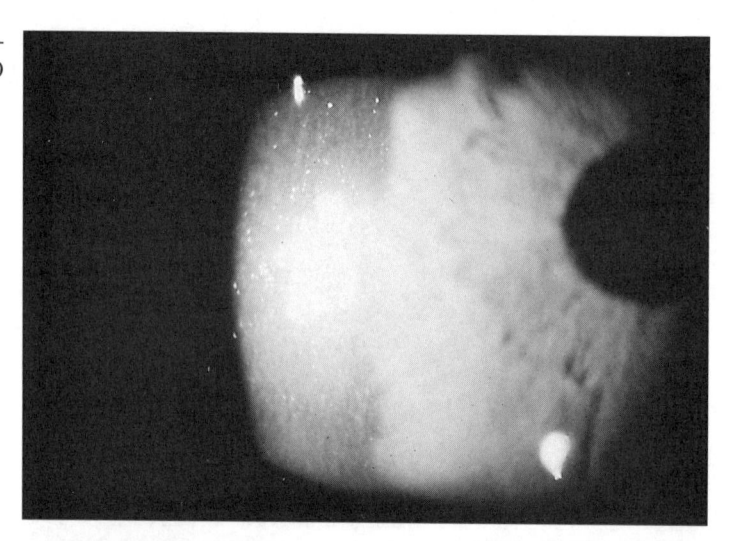

Figure 9-17. Corneal ulcer. (Photograph courtesy of EL Hargis, MD.)

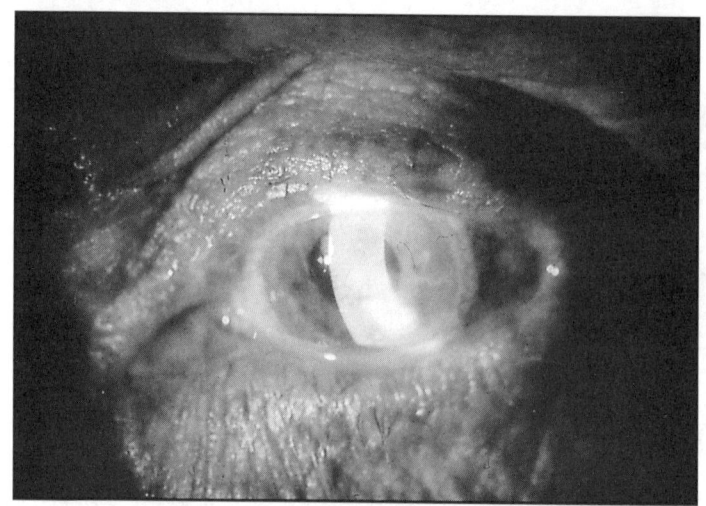

(Figure 9-18). If left untreated, the ulceration may spread into the stroma causing scarring, decreased vision, and intraocular infection. Symptoms include redness, pain or an FB sensation, tearing, and light sensitivity. Treatment includes anti-viral medications.

Herpes zoster is produced by the same virus that causes chicken pox. The virus becomes active and travels down nerve fibers of some parts of the body. It produces a blistering skin rash (shingles), fever, and painful inflammation of the affected nerve fibers. The virus may travel to the head and neck and can involve the eye, nose, mouth, cheek, and forehead. The virus infects the cornea in about 40% of those with shingles in the facial area. The infection causes corneal inflammation and lesions that can invade the stroma and cause scarring if left untreated. Treatment is early use of antiviral medications.

Bacteria, usually Staphylococcus aureus, can cause marginal corneal ulcers that extend from the limbus onto the cornea from 2 to 4 mm. There is marked redness, pain, and discharge. Treatment is usually with antibiotic and steroidal medications.

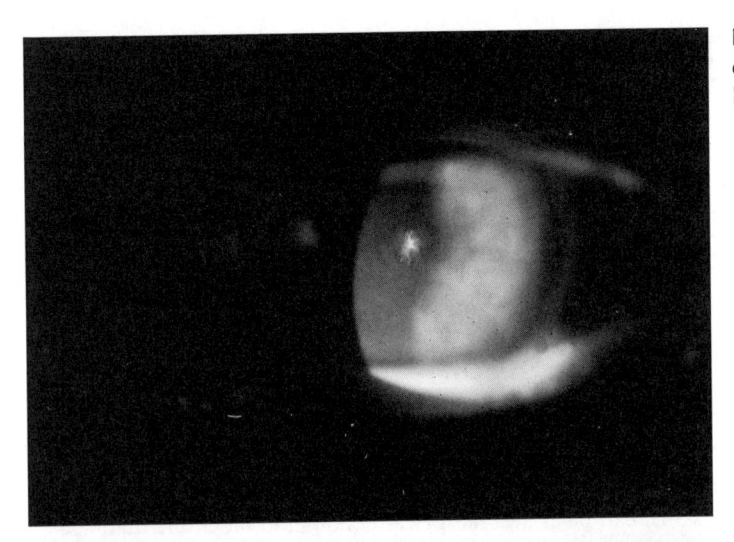

Figure 9-18. Herpetic dendrite. (Photograph courtesy of EL Hargis, MD.)

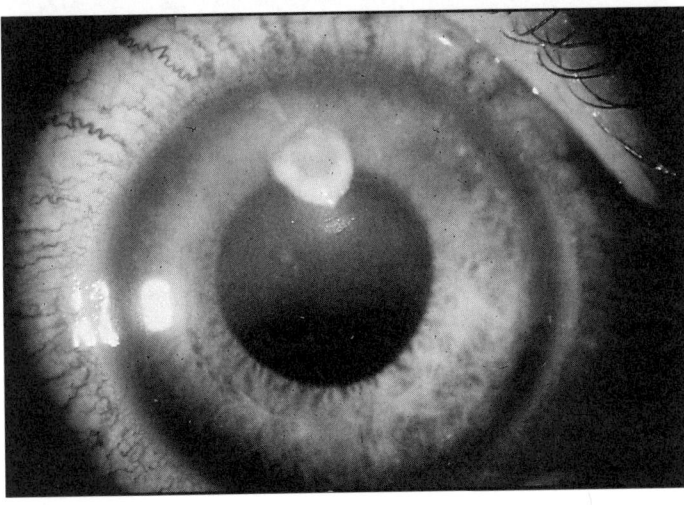

Figure 9-19. Soft contact lens-related keratitis. (Photograph courtesy of TD Lindquist, MD, PhD.)

Keratitis From Other Sources

Keratitis may result from contact lens overwear (Figure 9-19). The patient removes his or her contact lenses and within several hours has severe eye pain with redness due to epithelial damage. Treatment is systemic analgesics and patching. This condition should clear up within 24 to 48 hours.

Excessive exposure to ultraviolet light, such as from a sun lamp or welding arc, is another source of keratitis. Symptoms and treatment are the same as for contact lens overwear.

Keratitis can also occur if acid or alkaline chemicals burn the cornea. Acid burns cause immediate surface damage. Alkali burns are more destructive, causing both immediate surface and delayed penetrating damage. Any chemical splash requires immediate irrigation for a minimum of 20 minutes before the patient ever comes to the office. Irrigation needs to continue once the patient arrives at the office. Chemical injuries are discussed in more detail in Chapter 4.

The Anterior Chamber

The anterior chamber of the eye is located behind the cornea and in front of the iris. This space is filled with aqueous humor, a clear fluid that is produced by the ciliary processes (behind the iris). This fluid flows over the back of the iris (in the posterior chamber) and through the pupil into the anterior chamber, and then leaves the eye through the trabecular meshwork in the anterior chamber angle. If these trabecular drainage channels become partially or totally blocked, the aqueous cannot exit. This causes a rise in IOP.

Primary Angle-Closure Glaucoma (PACG)

An attack of PACG is brought on by a sudden rise in IOP due to anterior segment angle-closure. Individuals with narrow angles (a physiologically short distance between the iris and the cornea) are most at risk. There is also a natural increase in lens size as we age. For those with narrow angles, this increase in lens size can push the iris forward enough to block the drainage channels. Other factors that can bring on an episode of angle-closure glaucoma (for those with narrow angles) are dilation drops, dim lights, emotional stress, and some topical or systemic drugs (typically those that cause some pupil dilation).

Symptoms of angle-closure glaucoma (also known as a glaucoma attack) include severe ocular pain or headache, blurred vision, halos around lights, and possibly nausea and vomiting. Signs include redness, a mid-dilated pupil, and a cloudy cornea. (In contrast, open-angle glaucoma is painless and does not produce ocular redness). IOP can rise to 60 mm of mercury or more in angle-closure glaucoma. If the high pressure continues, optic nerve damage occurs, resulting in permanent vision loss. This is why angle-closure glaucoma is an emergency. Treatment is aimed at bringing the pressure down rapidly and can consist of the use of pilocarpine (a miotic) to constrict the pupil and pull the iris away from the cornea. Topical drops, such as levobunolol and dorozolamide, may be used to lower the pressure along with oral osmotics (such as glycerol mixed with fruit juice) or intravenous osmotics (such as mannitol). The osmotic agents draw water from the eye and thus work to reduce the pressure.

Hyphema and Hypopyon

A hypopyon is a pool of pus that forms at the bottom of the anterior chamber due to infection or inflammation within the eye, and may be associated with ocular redness (Figure 9-20).

A hyphema is a pool of blood that forms at the bottom of the anterior chamber as the result of trauma or disease (Figure 9-21). Treatment for these conditions depend on the cause, and should be seen on an emergent basis.

The Uveal Tract

The uveal tract consists of the iris, the ciliary body, and the choroid.

Anterior Uveitis (Iritis)

Anterior uveitis (also referred to as iritis) is an inflammation of the iris (Figure 9-22). Usually it appears without a known cause, although it may be related to systemic diseases such as arthritis, lupus, psoriasis, sarcoidosis, or ulcerative colitis. Symptoms are similar to acute glau-

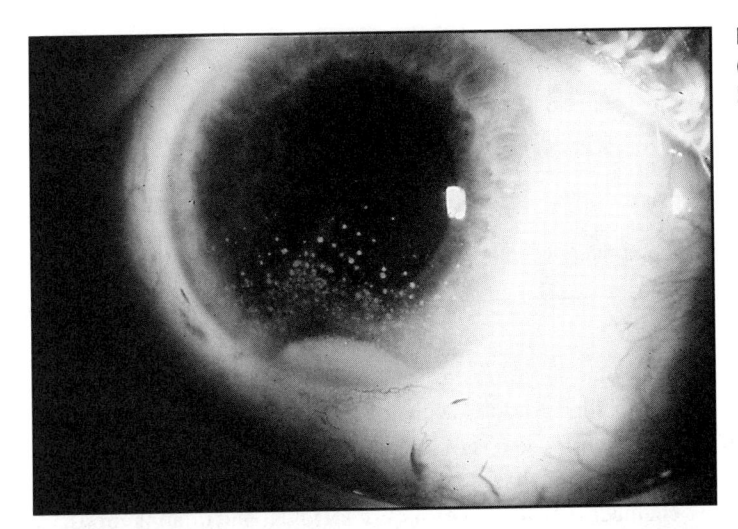

Figure 9-20. Hypopyon. (Photograph courtesy of Paula Parker, COMT.)

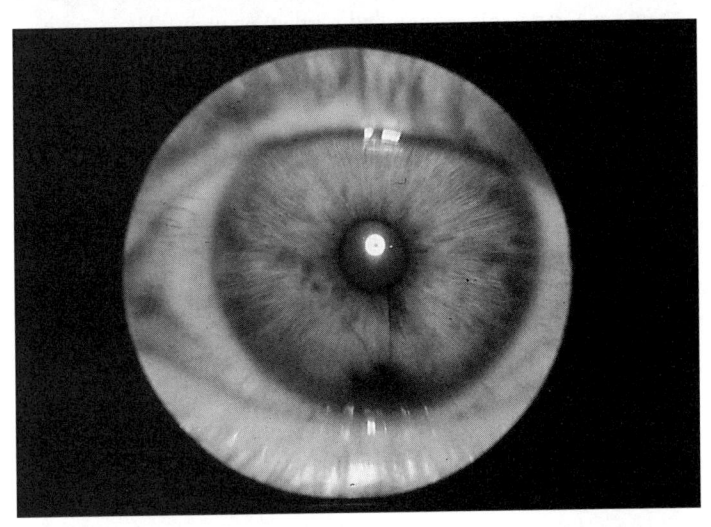

Figure 9-21. Hyphema. (Photograph courtesy of the Virginia Mason Medical Center.)

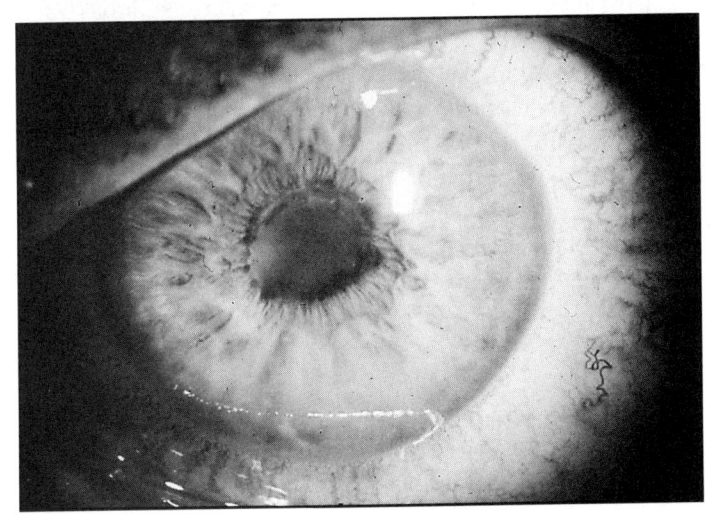

Figure 9-22. Iritis. (Photograph courtesy of TD Lindquist, MD, PhD.)

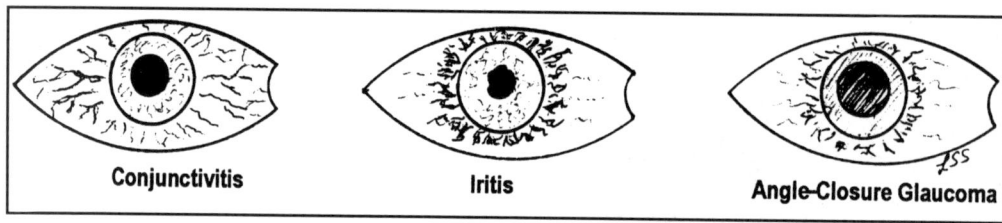

Figure 9-23. Schematic comparison of conjunctivitis, iritis, and angle-closure glaucoma. (Illustration by LS Sims, COT.)

coma, which include ocular redness, pain, blurred vision, tearing, and light sensitivity. However, the pupil of the affected eye is generally smaller, while in acute glaucoma the pupil is mid-dilated (Figure 9-23 and Table 9-1). The associated redness is often located at the limbus (termed ciliary flush) instead of the diffuse redness of conjunctivitis. A critical sign for diagnosis is the presence of cells and flare in the anterior chamber. Treatment consists of steroidal and dilating drops. Iritis (along with its treatment) can cause cataracts, glaucoma, and corneal changes. The patient who has a previous iritis episode tends to recognize the symptoms in the early stages of onset and seek treatment.

Posterior Uveitis

Posterior uveitis is an inflammation of the choroid due to conditions such as toxoplasmosis (infection of the body tissue by the Toxoplasma gondii protozoan, which can cause retinal and choroidal inflammation and scarring), sarcoidosis (an inflammatory condition of unknown origin that infects all body systems with microscopic nodules), syphilis (a venereal disease that in its late stages can affect the optic nerve, cause retinal vascularization, keratitis, uveitis, and vitritis), pars planitis (inflammation of the ciliary body in the pars plana region that leads to debris in the vitreous), ocular histoplasmosis (a fungal infection commonly found in the Ohio-Mississippi river valley area that occurs from inhaling Histoplasma capsulatum and can affect the optic nerve area, choroid and macula years later). Other causes can be trauma, surgery, or a weakened immune system from such conditions as chemotherapy treatment or acquired immunodeficiency syndrome (AIDS). Often, however, the cause is unknown. Posterior uveitis can lead to glaucoma, cataract formation, choroidal neovascularization, or RD. Signs and symptoms include pain, possible decreased vision, redness, light sensitivity, floaters, and a constricted pupil. Critical signs for diagnosis is the presence of white blood cells and opacities in the vitreous (vitritis), and retinal or choroidal infiltrates and edema. Patients presenting with such symptoms should be seen on an urgent basis. Treatment is dependent on the cause but can include dilation to prevent the lens from sticking to the iris (posterior synechiae) and the use of steroids by either topical, systemic, or retrobulbar routes to reduce inflammation.

The Vitreous

The vitreous is the clear gel-like substance that fills the posterior segment between the lens and the retina.

Table 9-1.
Red Eye Differential Diagnosis

	Conjunctivitis	Iritis	Acute Angle-Closure Glaucoma	Keratitis/ Corneal FB
Vision	Normal to blurring that clears with blinking	Mild blurring	Considerable blurring or haziness; halos around lights	Mild blurring
Pain	None to minor discomfort, burning or grittiness	Moderate to severe aching	Severe aching	Sharp pain or FB sensation
Discharge	Dependent on type: Mucopurulent—Bacterial Watery—Viral Watery/stringy—Allergic	None	None	None to mild
Pattern of Redness	Palpebral conjunctiva and/or diffuse bulbar conjunctiva	Conjunctival-circumcorneal pattern	Diffuse conjunctiva with prominent circumcorneal pattern	Conjunctival-circumcorneal pattern
Pupils	Normal, reactive	Constricted-may be slightly reactive	Dilated, fixed	Normal to constricted, reactive
Cornea	Clear	Clear to slightly hazy	Hazy	Possible visible FB opacification, abnormal light reflex, fluorescein staining
IOP	Normal	Normal to low	High	Normal
Other		Photophobia	Possible nausea and vomiting	Possible photophobia

Endophthalmitis

Endophthalmitis is an infection of the vitreous and surrounding tissues following surgery or injury. It is an emergency situation, as the infection can destroy the eye within days. Posterior endophthalmitis typically occurs within 2 to 4 days after surgery, although onset can be much later. Signs and symptoms include redness, corneal haze, pain, reduced vision, and sometimes a hypopyon. Treatment is massive doses of systemic and local antibiotics. Surgical removal of the vitreous (vitrectomy) is sometimes required.

Review of History and Triage

OptA

A well-gathered history can be very helpful to the physician. Primary questions to ask the patient presenting with ocular redness include:
- When did the redness start? (As a general rule, the more recent the onset, the more urgent the problem.)

- Is it getting worse?
- Is the eye also painful?
- Have you noticed any vision changes?
- Is there any discharge? What is the appearance of the discharge? Is it clear and thin, or thick and colored? If colored, is it white or yellow?
- Is the problem in one eye or both? If only in one eye, how is your vision in the non-affected eye?
- Have you had any recent surgery or injury to the eye?
- Have you had similar previous episodes?
- Do other members of your family have similar symptoms?
- Are you using any eye medication?
- Do you wear contact lenses?
- Do you have any preexisting eye problems, such as glaucoma?
- Do you have any preexisting medical problems?

Chapter 10

First Aid and Office Emergencies

OptA
OphA

Linda Sims, COT

KEY POINTS

- Every employee should regularly update his or her basic first aid skills and cardiopulmonary resuscitation (CPR) certification.

- Every person working in the office, regardless of his or her position, needs to know where the crash cart is kept.

- Someone should be assigned the duty of checking the cart every month to make sure that all supplies are present, in good condition, and unexpired.

- Everyone in the office needs to know the emergency response phone numbers, whether it be 911 for an external response team or an internal number for larger facilities who have their own emergency response teams.

A medical emergency can be defined as an injury or a sudden illness that requires immediate treatment to prevent death or organ damage. In a broader interpretation, a medical emergency can be any change in a person's medical status that is indicative of a deterioration of his or her condition or any unexpected occurrence (such as unconsciousness) that requires immediate attention.

Office Preparation for Emergencies

Although medical emergencies rarely occur, we need to be prepared to act quickly and appropriately when one does take place. Every employee in the office needs to know where the emergency supplies are located and how to assist in an emergency. Every employee should also regularly update his or her basic first aid skills and cardiopulmonary resuscitation (CPR) certification.

Emergency Cart

An emergency cart, also commonly referred to as a crash cart, is a portable cart or container that is stocked with items needed in times of emergency (Figure 10-1). Each clinic has its own specific needs as to the size and contents of a crash cart. A clinic that is located in a hospital will have different needs and requirements than a small, individual office.

Items commonly found in a crash cart include:
- Items for establishing an intravenous line, such as intravenous needles and tubing, tourniquets, alcohol wipes, tape, gauze, scissors, and intravenous solution bags such as dextrose and saline
- Items used for suction, such as suction tips, tubing, catheters, a lubricating jelly (to facilitate tube insertion) and a suction machine
- Items used to restore respiration, such as oxygen masks, barrier masks, nasal cannulas, bite blocks (used when the tongue starts to occlude the airway), and an oxygen tank
- Other miscellaneous items such as a blood pressure cuff and stethoscope, gloves, a sharps container, and various drugs such as epinephrine and diphenhydramine. An ophthalmic office may also wish to include bottled eye wash, a bottle of topical anesthetic (unopened, to ensure sterility), a lid speculum, and sterile cotton-tipped applicators.

All persons working in the office, regardless of their position, need to know where the crash cart is kept and be familiar with its contents in case they are called upon to assist in an emergency. Someone should be assigned the duty of checking the cart every month to make sure that all supplies are present, in good condition, and unexpired.

General Emergency Procedures

Assessment

In any emergency, start by assessing the person's life support functions.
- Is the person's airway occluded? Remove any obstruction to open the airway.
- Is the person breathing? Look for chest expansions, listen and feel for exhaled air. If breathing cannot be detected, begin rescue breathing.

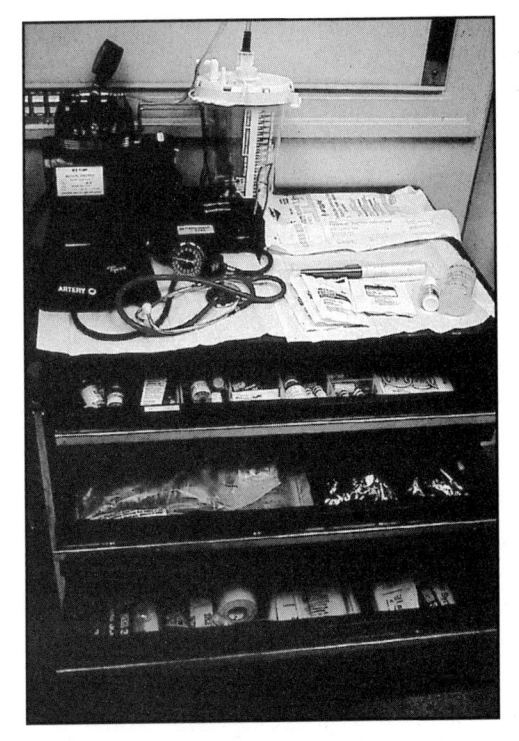

Figure 10-1. Emergency cart. (Photograph courtesy of LS Sims, COT.)

- Is the person's heart beating? Check the carotid pulse in an adult or child, or the brachial pulse in an infant. If you can't locate a pulse, start chest compressions. (For more information on clearing airway occlusions, rescue breathing, and administering chest compressions, see Chapter 11.)

Once you have ascertained that the patient is breathing and has a heartbeat, notify the physician of the occurrence and turn your attention to the patient's chief problem (see specific emergency situations later in this chapter). Question the patient or a family member about any known health conditions, medications, or allergies. Also check for a medical identification necklace or bracelet.

Remember that the patient and any family members present will be experiencing some level of anxiety. While a small amount of anxiety can sharpen a person's attention span, a moderate to high level of anxiety may decrease the person's attention and understanding, making them confused and uncooperative. Be prepared to offer reassurance and emotional support, and keep the environment calm and quiet. Maintain eye contact when speaking to the person, and keep your explanations as clear and simple as possible.

It is important to offer emotional support without giving any reassurance that can be construed as a medical guarantee. For example, if you tell a patient or family member, "Don't worry, everything will be alright," and everything *doesn't* turn out alright, you could be in legal trouble for implying that the outcome would be better. It is safer (and just as reassuring) to say, "Dr. Hubbard will do everything he can for you."

Also keep in mind that other healthcare workers may be functioning at less than optimal performance levels due to the stress of the situation. Keep communications as clear and precise as possible and double-check any orders that are unclear.

Feeling Faint and Fainting

Fainting (syncope) occurs due to insufficient oxygen reaching the brain resulting in temporary loss of consciousness. The patient may report feeling dizzy, nauseated, and/or weak, and feel a need to lie down. If the patient is standing, immediately assist him or her to a sitting position to avoid a fall. Once the patient is seated, have him or her place the head between the knees. If the patient is lying down, raise the feet. These two maneuvers will help blood get to the head, and may prevent fainting. Recovery from fainting will occur when normal blood flow to the brain is restored.

A fainting person usually falls or simply crumples to the ground. A patient who has already fainted is obviously unconscious, but may twitch or jerk slightly. When encountering a person who is unconscious, first check to see that he or she is breathing and has a pulse. If there is no pulse or respiration, start appropriate CPR procedures (see Chapter 11). If the person does have a pulse and is breathing, elevate the legs, loosen the collar or other tight clothing, and immediately notify the doctor of the occurrence. Smelling salts or aromatic spirits of ammonia may be used to help stimulate breathing by reflex. The person should remain lying down for 10 to 15 minutes after regaining consciousness. Reassure the patient, who may feel disoriented or embarrassed by the incident, and be prepared to steady the patient when he or she stands.

One common cause of fainting encountered in a medical office is known as a vasovagal attack, which occurs when the vagus nerve (that helps to control breathing and circulation of the blood) is overstimulated due to stress, fear, or pain. A vasovagal episode is usually accompanied by profuse sweating and paleness of the skin. In eyecare, such activities as instilling eyedrops, inserting a contact lens, or having applanation tonometry may precipitate a vasovagal response resulting in fainting. The patient who has had surgery (including minor procedures such as chalazion excision, cryopexy, or laser treatment) may faint as an emotional response to the procedure.

Fainting may also occur after standing still for long periods or from suddenly standing after sitting. This happens due to blood pooling in the veins of the legs, which reduces the amount of blood available to be pumped to the brain and results in a drop in blood pressure (postural hypotension). Postural hypotension more commonly occurs in the elderly, diabetics, and persons taking antihypertensive and vasodilator drugs. Any patient who is reclining should be encouraged to sit up slowly and remain seated for several moments.

Other causes of fainting are transient ischemic attacks (in which there is a temporary obstruction of blood flow to the brain), arrhythmia (an irregularity of the heartbeat), heart attack, stroke, or shock.

Shock

Physical shock occurs when there is a massive reduction of blood flow throughout the body tissues, leading to a lack of oxygen to the brain. This in turn affects the nervous system, allowing the blood vessels to become over-dilated and unresponsive. As the blood vessels enlarge, blood pressure drops further, leading to a downward spiral from which the body cannot recover on its own. If there is no intervention, death occurs.

A decrease in blood flow can occur for various reasons. Cardiogenic shock occurs when the heart is not pumping out a sufficient quantity of blood. This may result from a sudden blockage of a blood vessel that leads to the heart (myocardial infarction, commonly known as a heart attack) or other conditions of myocardial ischemia (where there is localized lack of blood).

Hypovolemic shock occurs when there is a large loss of blood or other body fluid to the point that there is insufficient blood in the body to maintain pressure. This can result from injury or from disorders such as a perforated ulcer, prolonged diarrhea, or injury.

Other types of shock occurs because the diameter of the blood vessels have become so enlarged that the blood supply is insufficient to maintain blood pressure, even though the actual volume of blood has not changed (anaphylactic and septic shock). Anaphylactic shock can be the result of an intense allergic reaction to foods, sulfites, insect venom (such as bee stings), medications such as penicillin, or injected substances (such as a rare reaction to fluorescein sodium used in fluorescein angiograms). Septic shock occurs as a result of a severe infection that spreads throughout the body via the blood stream.

The symptoms of shock include sweating, rapid/shallow breathing, rapid but weak pulse, cold moist skin, dizziness, weakness, and fainting. A conscious person who is in shock may become thirsty, anxious, confused, and drowsy.

Emergency treatment for shock includes maintaining an open airway, CPR if breathing and heart beat stops, elevating the legs (to promote blood to move from the legs to the head and central organs), and reducing heat loss with blankets. (However, if the person has symptoms of a heart attack such as chest pain, or trouble breathing, do not place him or her on the back. Instead, ease breathing by raising him or her to a half-sitting position.) Do not administer food or drink until an emergency team or doctor has evaluated the person.

Immediately call the physician, 911, or your emergency response team (if your facility is so equipped). Treatment by the doctor or emergency response team may include injection of epinephrine (which frees breathing passages and stimulates the cardiovascular system), diazepam (for seizures), diphenhydramine (an anti-histamine that counteracts the histamines released as the result of an allergic reaction), or intravenous steroids (to decrease swelling and itching). Administration of oxygen, intravenous fluid, or blood transfusions, and injections of painkillers such as morphine may also be necessary. Once blood pressure is restored, treatment will be directed at the underlying condition that brought on the shock. Full recovery usually depends on the underlying cause and the swiftness and effectiveness of the emergency treatment given during the crucial minutes that the body was in shock.

Insulin Shock

Insulin is a hormone that helps convert food into energy. In diabetes mellitus, the body's ability to maintain the correct proportion of insulin and glucose is impaired and throws off the normal balance, resulting in either a too high (hyperglycemia), or a too low (hypoglycemia) level of blood glucose. Insulin shock occurs when there is a low level of blood glucose and a high level of insulin in the body.

Insulin shock can lead to an extreme decrease in blood pressure (hypotension), a decrease of blood flow to organs, coma, and death.

Causes of insulin shock in a diabetic include not eating properly (resulting in the body not getting enough sugar), excessive exercising (which affects the amount of sugar the body needs for maintenance), taking the incorrect amount of insulin, and not preparing the insulin properly.

Signs and symptoms of insulin shock include a change in personality (such as aggression or confusion), dizziness, trembling, cold moist skin, hunger, salivation, headache, rapid but weak pulse, seizures, and loss of consciousness.

Treatment for insulin shock must be given by an emergency response team or a physician, who will start a glucagon or dextrose intravenous line. Call for help immediately any time a patient becomes unconscious. Until help arrives, make sure the patient's airway is clear, and that he or she is breathing and has a pulse. (Start CPR if necessary.) Never attempt to give an unconscious person food or drink.

Treatment for a conscious person going into insulin shock includes oral administration of a glucose product if available, a glass of fruit juice (such as orange or apple), a soft drink containing sugar (ie, not a diet drink), sugar water, or corn syrup. We will often know that the patient is a diabetic, but we will not know if the insulin reaction they are experiencing is due to hypoglycemia or hyperglycemia. Your first course of action should be to alert the physician, who can make such medical decisions. If there is no other help available, activate the emergency medical system (dial 911).

Seizures

A seizure is defined as a sudden episode of uncontrolled electrical energy in the brain. If this abnormal energy in the brain is confined to one area, the person may only have slight tingling or twitching in one area of the body. (Other symptoms can include hallucinations or feelings of fear or familiarity.) If the entire brain is affected by the abnormal electrical activity, the person loses consciousness (a grand mal seizure). Recurrent seizures are referred to as epilepsy.

A seizure sometimes occurs without known reason. However there are a number of known causes, some of which include arsenic or lead poisoning, brain abscesses or tumors, meningitis, stroke, electrolyte abnormalities, hypoglycemia, multiple sclerosis, sarcoidosis, and Sturge-Weber syndrome.

Regardless of the cause, your main goal during a seizure is to keep the patient from harming him or herself. Place a pillow or other soft material under the head. Loosen any tight clothing and move any hard or sharp objects out of the way. Stay with the patient; do not try to restrain the person. Do not try to hold the patient's mouth open or place your fingers inside the mouth.

During the tonic phase of a seizure, the person's muscles contract, the body stiffens, eyelids open, and the mouth opens wide and then snaps shut. (This is why you should not put fingers or other objects into the patient's mouth). The next phase, the clonic phase, starts with mild trembling and progresses to violent jerking movements and spewing of foamy, bloody saliva. At the end of this phase, turn the patient on his side to allow secretions to drain from the mouth. If respiration does not resume, check the patient's airway for obstruction, as these secretions sometimes block the airway.

During the recovery phase, the patient will be confused, disoriented, and very tired. Stay with the patient, offer reassurance, and provide a quiet place for him or her to rest. Record information such as time and duration of seizure, any unusual occurrences prior to the seizure (such as reported auras or mood changes), what happened during the seizure (such as type of muscle movements and whether consciousness was lost), and what occurred after the seizure (such as patient confusion, grogginess, or even remembering the seizure).

When a seizure starts, activate the emergency system. When assistance arrives, an IV line and airway may be started as necessary. The patient may receive anti-convulsive medications and be put on a cardiac monitor, as needed.

Falls

Falls at the office can happen at any time. Some falls occur from a medical condition which leaves the person weak, dizzy, or feeling off-balance. Other falls may occur as a result of fainting, seizures, or shock. Some falls are purely accidental, such as tripping over a chair or electrical cord, or as a result of poor lighting making obstacles harder to see, especially for persons with decreased vision.

If you are with the person when they begin to fall, try to break the fall with your body while gently guiding him or her to the floor. If you are near a wall, gently guide the person toward the wall and allow him or her to slide down the wall while offering as much support as you can manage. Remember to keep your feet apart to give yourself a better center of gravity and thus more balance. Also, bend your knees, not your back, to avoid injuring yourself while trying to soften the fall.

If you come upon a person who has fallen, assess the situation before allowing the patient to move or stand. Ask the person or a witness what occurred. Did the patient lose consciousness or experience pain? Try to determine the extent of any injuries such as lacerations, abrasions, or broken bones.

Notify the doctor and try to keep the patient still and comfortable until the doctor examines him or her. Use blankets and pillows for comfort, unless a spinal cord injury is suspected, in which case do *not* elevate the head with a pillow. Spinal cord injuries as a result of a fall are rare, but if present, any movement can result in irreversible damage.

When it has been determined it is safe to move the patient, have a co-worker help if lifting is required. Attempting to lift a patient alone can result in injury to the patient or yourself.

Most facilities have incident reports that must be filled out in the event of any accident occurring on the premises. Be aware of the requirements of your facility and file the appropriate reports.

Drug Reactions

When speaking of basic first aid, we need to keep in mind that many of the medications administered in the eyecare setting (in topical, injected, or oral form) may cause side effects or allergic reactions in some patients. Most of these side effects or allergies are minor, but others may be life-threatening.

An allergy is a by-product of an immune system response triggered by a foreign substance. The immune response is the body's attempt to detect and eliminate the foreign substance. During this response, the body releases substances such as histamines, which cause the allergic symptoms of swelling, redness, and itching.

Some of the more commonly used general and ophthalmic medications are listed in this chapter. Many ophthalmic medications are derivatives of drugs that produce common allergic reactions in the general population, such as sulfa, the "cillins" (penicillin), the "caines"(cocaine), and steroids. When obtaining or updating a patient history, be sure to review and record current known allergies.

If a patient has an immediate response to a topically applied medication in the eyecare office, notify the doctor. If the reaction is strictly local (redness and itching) it will most likely be alleviated by thoroughly irrigating the eye(s) with an eye wash or saline solution. Follow your doctor's instructions and document the medication, type of reaction, and the action(s) taken.

Sulfa and Derivatives

Sulfa and its derivatives are broad spectrum antimicrobial drugs that produce an allergic reaction in approximately 5 to 10% of the population. Allergic reactions include nausea, vomiting, headaches, dizziness, fever, and rash.

Ophthalmic use is primarily via topical solutions and ointments containing sulfacetamide and oral carbonic anhydrase inhibitors (CAI's) such as acetazolamide and methazolamide.

Topical reactions include swelling, redness, vesiculation (blisters), and scaling. Sensitizations may recur when a sulfa drug is readministered regardless of the route. CAI allergic reactions include fever, rash, damage to blood cell production, and rare cases of fatality if the reaction is severe. Toxic reactions include tingling, nausea, anorexia, weight loss, fatigue, and kidney stones.

Penicillin and Derivatives

Penicillin is a common antibiotic to which 1 to 10% of the population is allergic. Allergic reactions can range from mild rash, fever, and nausea, to swelling, throat and breathing tube spasms, chills, fever, and anaphylactic shock (see Shock, this chapter).

Anesthetics

Cocaine is a naturally occurring compound that has a topical anesthetic effect. It is rarely used as an ophthalmic anesthetic because it causes corneal epithelial damage, produces pupil dilation, and may affect IOP. Because of its actions on the cornea, it is sometimes used in corneal debridement for dendritic keratitis.

Other "caine" drugs are synthetic compounds, such as proparacaine hydrochloride (which can also be found in some fluorescein drops), tetracaine hydrochloride, and lidocaine.

Allergic side effects include decreased blood pressure, decreased breathing, and seizures. Allergies to topically applied anesthetics are infrequent and usually are limited to skin reactions.

Fluorescein Dyes

Fluorescein dyes are diagnostic drugs that glow under a cobalt blue light. Topical fluorescien is used to observe corneal irregularities and to take applanation tonometry readings. It can also be injected intravenously to photograph the blood flow in the retina.

Topical allergies to fluorescein drops are uncommon. When used as an injection, severe anaphylactic allergic reactions can occur, although this is rare. Allergic reactions from injection can include an itching skin rash, difficulty breathing, swelling of the larynx, a rapid and weak pulse, and circulatory collapse. (See Shock, this chapter).

Steroids

Steroids are derivatives of the adrenal hormone cortisone, and can be given topically, orally, or by injection. Some common steroids are hydrocortisone, prednisolone, dexamethasone, and progesterone-like compounds (such as medrysone and fluorometdoctrine). Steroids reduce inflammation, redness, swelling, and scarring by slowing the body's battle against foreign substances or itself. Because it slows the body's fighting responses, it can actually worsen certain infections such as herpes simplex and fungal infections. Other side effects include decreased wound healing, cataract formation, and glaucoma. Diabetes, weakness, and high blood pressure can result from oral administration.

Beta Blockers

Beta blockers are a class of drugs that block the action of the sympathetic nervous system and are commonly used to treat glaucoma. Betaxolol, levobunolol, metipranolol, timolol, and dorazolamide are all examples of beta blockers.

Allergic reactions and side effects can include congestive heart failure, bronchiospasm and worsening of asthma, depression, impotence, fatigue, and masking of hypoglycemic symptoms (in diabetics).

Basic First Aid for Ocular Emergencies

Ocular emergencies are usually the result of chemical burns, penetrating injuries, CRAOs, blunt trauma, FBs, acute glaucoma attacks, or sudden onset of pain without known cause. The three cases needing treatment within minutes are chemical burns of the eye, penetrating injuries to the eye, and a sudden painless loss of vision (a possible CRAO). Other cases need to be seen within hours, but the sooner we can see the patient, the easier the exam may be and the better the prognosis may be.

While all ocular emergencies must be treated by a doctor, we need to be aware of what we should and should not do in the event of an ocular emergency:

- Do have the proper emergency supplies on hand and readily accessible.
- Do have sterile (unopened) eyedrops and ointments on hand for use when dealing with a traumatized eye (however, do not use until instructed to do so by the physician).
- Do lightly patch the eye and get assistance if uncertain what to do. The exception to patching is with a chemical splash or protruding FB.
- Do continue the irrigation process for any chemical splash patient immediately upon arrival for a period of at least 20 minutes. (The patient should have started this process before coming to your office.)
- Do tell the patient that the doctor will do everything possible to help him or her.
- Do not tell the patient that "everything will be all right."
- Do not put pressure on a traumatized eye.
- Do not instill eye medications unless instructed to do so by the physician.
- Do not use any ophthalmic instruments on a traumatized eye.

Sudden, Painless Loss of Vision

A sudden, painless loss of vision may indicate a CRAO, which must be treated within minutes if the eyesight is to be saved. There is nothing that we, as eyecare assistants, can do for the patient except to get him or her in to see a physician as quickly as possible. If the patient is phoning in to report the problem, have him or her come in immediately and alert the front desk assistants and the doctor that the patient is on the way. Get the patient in to see the physician immediately upon arrival. Patients who have a long distance to travel to arrive at your office should go to an emergency room near their home.

The ophthalmologist may perform paracentesis (a procedure during which a sharp object is passed through the anterior chamber in an attempt to quickly lower IOP, which may cause some blood to flow back into the retinal artery, allowing the obstruction to pass).

Other possible causes of a sudden, painless loss of vision include RDs, vitreous hemorrhage, or CRVO, which should be seen within hours. (See Chapter 8.)

The Patient in Pain

A sudden onset of eye pain can result from many ocular problems. A dull ache will usually indicate a problem within the eye, while a sharp stabbing pain is more indicative of a corneal problem.

Ascertain if any trauma has occurred (blunt trauma, an FB, or penetrating injury), if the patient has had recent ocular surgery or a history of corneal transplant surgery, if there is a history of glaucoma, iritis, or other ocular disease, or if the patient is a contact lens wearer. Do not base an evaluation of the situation by the severity of pain alone. Deep, penetrating injuries can be less painful than a superficial corneal abrasion.

Signs and symptoms such as visual acuity, redness, tearing, discharge, swelling, pupil reflexes, and the possibility of trauma must also be taken into consideration.

If trauma has not occurred, check the patient's visual acuity, pupil responses, and intraocular pressure, if appropriate. If trauma has occurred, do not touch the eye, notify the doctor immediately, and follow his or her instructions. In any case, do not instill any eyedrops or administer any pain medications unless instructed to do so by the physician.

Trauma

Ocular trauma is any injury to the eye. In blunt trauma an object strikes the eye but does not penetrate it (such as a fist, racquetball, baseball bat, or hammer). A penetrating injury occurs when a foreign object penetrates the globe. This can occur from high velocity missiles hitting the eye during carpentry work, yard maintenance, automobile accidents, etc, and can include objects such as wood particles, wire, and glass. A frequent cause of trauma is from surface FBs that may be imbedded in the cornea or conjunctiva but have not penetrated the globe. Contact lenses may cause corneal abrasions, which can lead to infection and ulceration if left untreated.

In any case of trauma, do *not* touch the eye. If the globe is perforated, any pressure on the eye may cause the contents of the globe to be expelled through the perforation. Suspect a penetration of the globe if lid lacerations are present. In the case of penetrating injuries, immediately notify the physician on the patient's arrival.

Depending on the severity of the trauma, attempt to obtain the patient's visual acuity (if possible), a description of the nature and time of the trauma, and any treatment prior to arriving at the office. Again, do not put any pressure on the eye and do not give any medications until instructed to do so by the ophthalmologist. To ensure sterility, use only unopened eye medications when dealing with a traumatized eye.

Chemical Splash

A patient who phones in stating that a chemical has gotten into the eye should be instructed to immediately irrigate the eye by holding it open under running tap water for a minimum of 15 to 20 minutes *before* coming into the office or emergency room.

The office person taking the initial phone call should notify the front desk, the back office assistants, and the doctor that a person with a chemical splash is coming in so that irrigation can continue immediately upon his or her arrival.

Once the patient arrives, continue to flush the eye with sterile saline solution or tap water for 20 to 30 minutes. The physician may want to insert a lid speculum to facilitate rinsing of the eye.

Items to have prepared for the patient's arrival include sterile saline (preferably in intravenous drip-type bags), intravenous tubing, an intravenous stand, sterile topical anesthetic (proparacaine), a lid speculum, litmus paper (to test for pH neutrality to determine if irrigation is complete), and towels.

Chemical burns can result from alkali-based products such as ammonia and other cleaning products, calcium hydroxide or lime (which is used in cement, mortar, and plaster); acid-based products such as car batteries or laboratory tests; or from organic solvents, such as kerosene, gasoline, or alcohol. (See Chapter 4 for more information on chemical burns.)

Managing Emergencies When the Doctor is Out

It may sometimes happen that an emergency will arise when the doctor is not on the premesis. Usually this comes as a phone call, with a patient telephoning about a potentially serious problem. First, you should follow the routine of phone triage as outlined in Chapter 1. (If the patient has come into the office, the triage questions may be asked in person, assisted by the fact that you can visually examine the patient.)

Before this situation arises, you should discuss with your physician as to how he or she wants you to handle such problems. Under what circumstances does he or she wish to be paged? Is there another eyecare practitioner in the area who will take call for your physician? (If so, the dates, names, and phone numbers should always be posted for reference.) Under what situations should you send the patient to the emergency room? Are there different guidelines for new patients versus established patients?

How far are you to go in offering care personally? Certainly you should irrigate a chemical splash, but how much farther should you go? Check an IOP? (Possibly.) Remove a corneal FB? (Doubtful!) These are medicolegal questions you should discuss with your physician. Then adhere to the rules.

Ideally, each of these issues should be in the office policy manual. In addition, it is vital to document any dealing with a patient, even if it is only over the phone. This is always true, but especially so when the doctor is not available. Write down the patient's name, the date and time of the phone call, the patient's complaint, your triage notes, and your recommendation as per office protocol.

Chapter 11

Cardiopulmonary Resuscitation

OphA

Leslie Hargis-Greenshields, COMT

KEY POINTS

- Basic life support includes the teaching of risk factors and the prevention of cardiac arrest by adopting a healthy lifestyle.
- CPR alone is not usually enough to save a life.
- Early activation of the emergency medical services (EMS) system is essential.
- The primary goal of CPR is to provide oxygen to the heart, brain, and other vital organs until advanced medical treatment can be applied.

CPR is just one component of emergency cardiac care (ECC). Each year thousands of lives are saved by prompt initiation of CPR. Because of the nature of our jobs in the healthcare environment, we need to be prepared to handle medical emergencies. Knowing the skills of CPR allows us to play an important role in ECC and situations of respiratory distress.

Emergency Cardiac Care

Emergency cardiac care is comprised of the following:
- Recognition of early warning signs of a heart attack.
- Immediate initiation of basic life support (BLS) at the scene.
- Starting advanced cardiac life support (ACLS) as quickly as possible, stabilizing the victim before transportation.
- Transfer of the victim to a hospital where advanced medical treatment can be provided.

BLS is the particular phase of ECC that either prevents circulatory or respiratory arrest through recognition and intervention or supports the victim of circulatory or respiratory arrest through CPR. In either case, a fast initiation of the emergency medical services (EMS) system is imperative.

Risk Factors and Prevention of Cardiac Arrest

BLS includes the teaching of risk factors and the prevention of cardiac arrest by adopting a healthy lifestyle.

Coronary artery disease affects the vessels that supply the heart with blood. Atherosclerosis is the buildup of fatty deposits on the artery walls and is the most common cause of coronary artery disease. This disease gradually narrows the arteries, which in turn decreases the blood flow. If the arteries of the heart are involved this could lead to a heart attack. If the arteries of the brain are involved this could lead to a stroke. In either case, the process of atherosclerosis usually begins at an early age. The development of atherosclerosis may be increased by a number of risk factors such as age, heredity, smoking, obesity, diabetes, high blood pressure, and lack of exercise.

Risk factors that cannot be changed:
- Heredity
- Age
- Race
- Gender

Risk factors that can be changed:
- High blood pressure
- High cholesterol
- Smoking
- Lack of exercise

Other contributing factors:
- Obesity
- Diabetes
- Increased stress

The danger of a heart attack increases with the number of risk factors present. By modifying lifestyle and decreasing the number of risk factors, the possibility of future heart disease may be minimized. Prudent heart living is the key to prevention.

Chain of Survival

CPR alone is usually not enough to save lives. Early activation of the EMS system and early CPR are essential in improving the survival and recovery rates of cardiac arrest victims. However, emergency cardiac care depends on a strong interaction between all four parts of the chain of survival. The chain of survival includes the following sequence:

- Early access into the EMS system (911)
- Early CPR
- Early defibrillation
- Early advanced care

Early Access to the EMS System

As soon as a medical emergency is recognized, the EMS system needs to be activated by calling 911 (Figure 11-1). This step is referred to as "phone first" and is used in situations where the victim is an adult. If you are alone, make the 911 call to activate the EMS system right away. This procedure is slightly modified to "phone fast" if the victim is a child. Since children generally suffer from conditions resulting in respiratory arrest (vs. cardiac arrest), it is important to give one minute of artificial respiration prior to activating the EMS system. Remember, "Phone first, phone fast." If a second rescuer is available, ask that person to first call for help and then return to the scene.

When you call 911, be prepared to tell the operator the following:

- The location of the emergency.
- What happened (ie, heart attack, car accident, drowning, etc).
- How many people are involved and their need of medical attention.
- What is currently being done for the victims, and their condition.
- Telephone number from which you are calling.

Early CPR

CPR externally supports the circulation and respiration of a victim of cardiac arrest through methods of artificial breathing and chest compressions. The primary goal of CPR is to provide oxygen to the heart, brain, and other vital organs until advanced medical treatment can be applied. Early CPR is the topic of this chapter.

The indications for CPR are respiratory arrest (in which respiration is externally supported) and cardiac arrest (in which both respiration and circulation are externally supported).

When breathing stops from conditions such as choking, drowning, stroke, heart attack, and drug overdose, the heart continues to pump blood for several minutes. This allows existing oxygen in the lungs and blood to continue to circulate to the brain and other organs for a short time. Early intervention of opening the airway and rescue breathing may prevent cardiac arrest.

Figure 11-1. Phone first, phone fast.

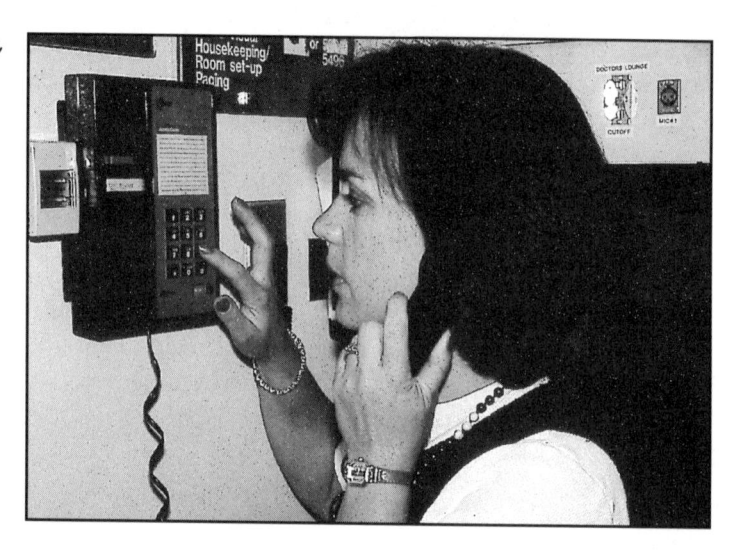

When the heart stops, blood is no longer circulated and oxygen in the vital organs is depleted in a matter of seconds. Prompt application of external chest compressions in combination with rescue breathing is necessary to prevent clinical death. Brain damage may begin 4 minutes after the heart stops; brain death occurs in approximately 10 minutes.

It is also prudent to know the signs and symptoms of a heart attack. They include:

- Chest discomfort (pressure, tightness, or pain that may radiate to shoulder, neck, lower jaw, or arms)
- Sweating
- Nausea
- Shortness of breath
- Weakness

Early Defibrillation

A defibrillator is a machine that delivers electric shocks to the heart. Early activation of the EMS system helps ensure that qualified emergency personnel will arrive quickly with the necessary equipment. In the case of an abnormal heart rhythm (one that prevents the heart from pumping blood) the earlier the shock from a defibrillator is delivered the more likely the victim can be saved.

Early Advanced Care

ACLS includes BLS plus the use of equipment, medications, cardiac monitoring, and post-resuscitation care. This specialized care requires the supervision of doctors as well as the support of nurses, paramedics, and other appropriately trained medical professionals.

CPR Procedure

The first step in CPR is to determine unresponsiveness. Assessing the unconscious victim is accomplished by shaking his or her shoulders gently and shouting, "Are you OK?" (Figure 11-2).

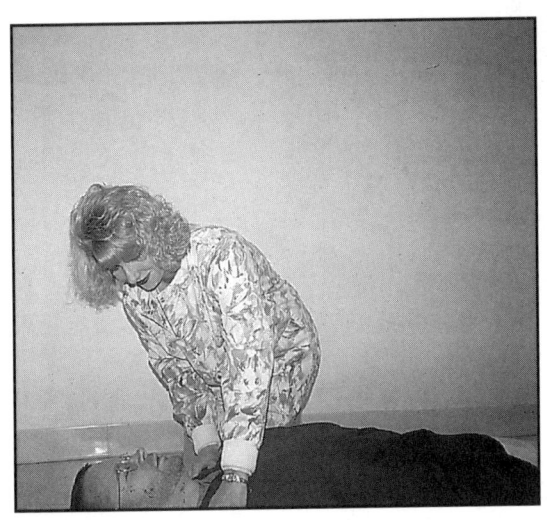

Figure 11-2. Shake and shout.

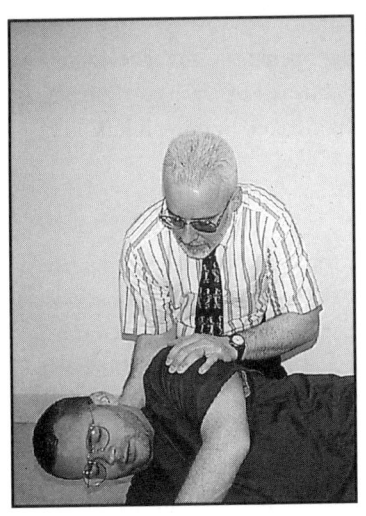

Figure 11-3. Position the victim by rolling him or her onto the back while supporting the head and neck.

The person who appears unconscious may just be sleeping or intoxicated. If the victim does not respond, consider him or her unconscious. Activate the EMS system as outlined earlier.

Position the victim by rolling him or her as a unit, onto the back while supporting the head and neck (Figure 11-3).

The ABC's of CPR

The techniques of CPR are similar whether a rescuer is performing CPR on a stroke victim, a pediatric resuscitation victim, or someone with an obstructed airway. These techniques include three basic skills that spell out the ABC's of CPR. They are airway, breathing, and circulation. (This section will give general instructions. Procedures for specific cases will follow.)

At the beginning of each of the ABC's of CPR is an assessment phase:

- Airway–determine unresponsiveness
- Breathing–determine breathlessness
- Circulation–determine if the person has a pulse

Figure 11-4. Head tilt/chin lift maneuver.

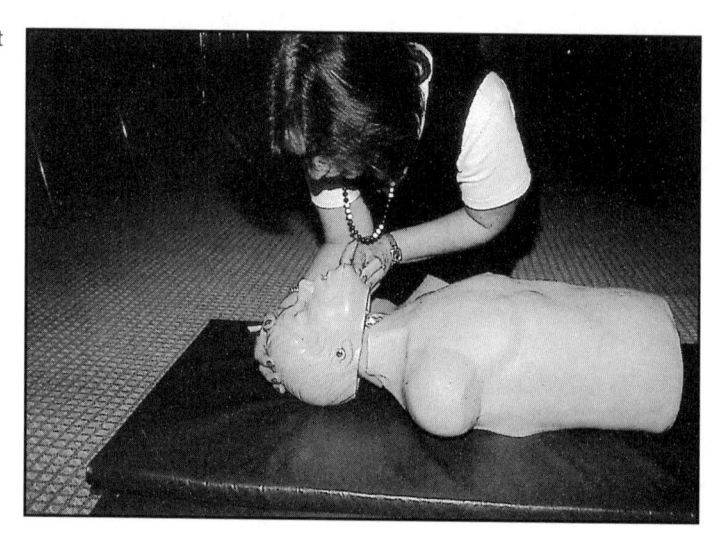

No victim should undergo any of the steps of CPR (positioning, opening of the airway, rescue breathing, or chest compressions) until the need has been established by each assessment. Never rehearse or practice the steps of CPR on a conscious healthy person. Serious injury may result if chest compressions are done on a beating heart.

Airway

After establishing the unresponsiveness of a victim, an airway must be established by properly positioning the head. The tongue and the epiglottis are the most common causes of obstructed airways in the unconscious victim. (Meat is the most common cause in the conscious victim.) Since the tongue is attached to the lower jaw, tilting the head back and moving the chin forward will usually open the airway. This is called the head tilt/chin lift maneuver (Figure 11-4). Place the fingers of one hand under the bony part of the victim's lower jaw. Care should be taken not to press on the soft tissue under the jaw. Place the other hand on the victim's forehead and press down to tilt the head back as the chin is lifted up. (It is incorrect to tilt the head by putting a hand under the victim's neck.)

Breathing

If breathing stops, the body has only enough oxygen remaining in the lungs and bloodstream to keep vital organs oxygenated for several minutes. Mouth-to-mouth rescue breathing is the fastest way to get oxygen into the victim's lungs. During rescue breathing the rescuer's exhaled air contains enough oxygen (roughly 16%) to support the victim.

To determine breathlessness, look, listen, and feel (Figure 11-5). Look at the chest for movement. Listen for sounds of breathing. Feel for breath on your cheek. If the victim is breathing, place him or her in the recovery position (Figure 11-6a and b). Using an arm and leg for stabilization, place the victim on his or her side. To roll the victim towards you, lift the victim's arm (closest to you) over the head and fold the far arm over the chest. Cross the far leg of the victim over the top of the other leg. Roll the victim as one unit towards you, taking care to support the head and neck.

If the victim is not breathing, pinch the nostrils closed and make a tight seal around the victim's mouth (Figure 11-7). Give two slow, full breaths (1.5 to 2 seconds per breath). Watch for the victim's chest to rise. If a tight seal cannot be made around the victim's mouth due to injury,

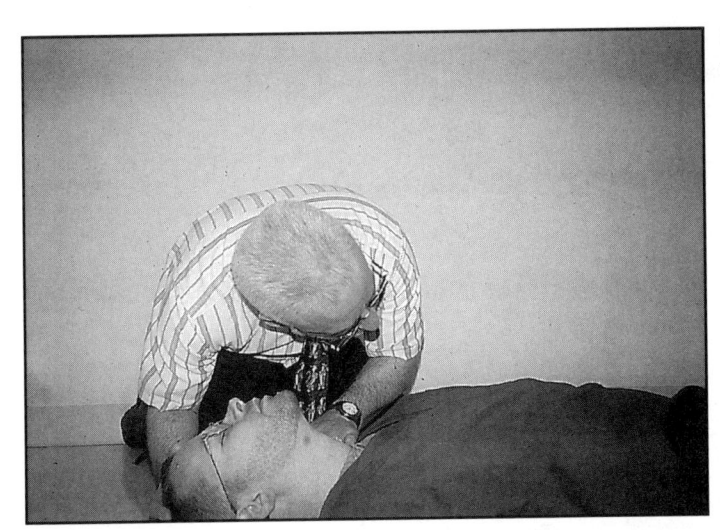

Figure 11-5. Look, listen, and feel for breathing.

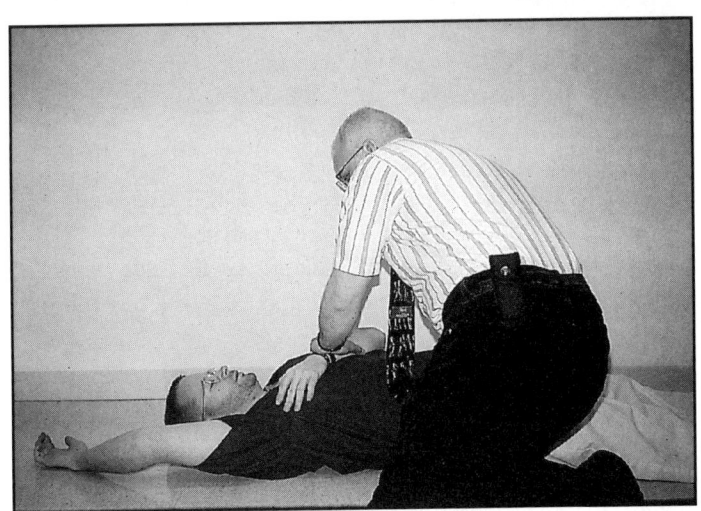

Figure 11-6a. Recovery position. Using an arm and a leg for stabilization, place the victim on his or her side. To roll the victim towards you, lift the victim's arm (closest to you) over the head and fold the far arm over the chest.

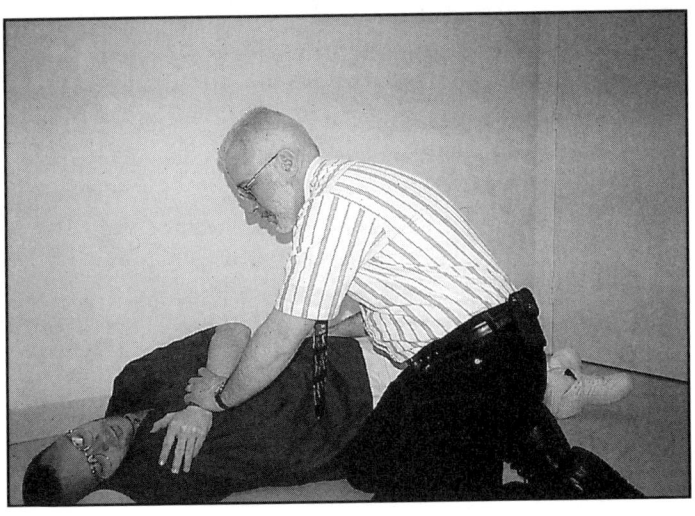

Figure 11-6b. Recovery position. Cross the far leg of the victim over the top of the other leg. Roll the victim towards you, taking care to support the head and neck.

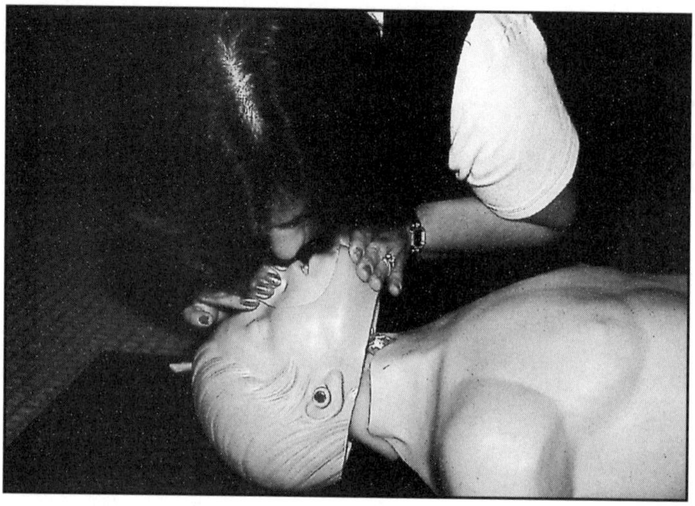

Figure 11-7. Pinch the nostrils closed and make a tight seal around the victim's mouth.

mouth-to-nose ventilation may be required. (Rates of breathing for adult and child and infant rescue will be given in a subsequent section.)

Circulation

Chest compressions can manually maintain some blood flow to the lungs, brain, and other major organs. When there is no pulse, chest compressions are necessary, as well as rescue breathing.

To determine if the person has a pulse, place 2 fingers on the Adam's apple. Slide fingers towards the floor into the indentation between the Adam's apple and the neck muscle. Check for the carotid pulse for 5 to 10 seconds (Figure 11-8).

If the victim has a pulse, continue rescue breathing at a rate of 1 breath every 5 seconds (or roughly 12 times per minute). If the victim has no pulse, begin the first set of chest compressions and ventilations. Position yourself at the victim's side. To find landmarks for proper hand position, follow the ribs up to the xiphoid process (or notch) where the ribs meet the sternum. Measure two fingers above the notch and place one hand on the lower half on the sternum (Figure 11-9). The first hand is removed from the notch and placed on top of the hand that rests on the sternum. Both hands should be parallel and directed away from the rescuer (Figure 11-10). The rescuer should lean forward to compress the chest with shoulders directly over the hands (Figure 11-11). In an adult, the sternum should be depressed 1.5 to 2 inches, at a rate of 80 to 100 compressions per minute. Counting is done to establish a rhythm such as "one and two and three and…" At the end of every 15 compressions, give 2 rescue breaths. Check to see if pulse has returned at the end of 4 cycles. If there is no pulse, resume CPR with 2 rescue breaths followed by 15 compressions. If there is a pulse, but no breathing, give one rescue breath every 5 seconds.

Procedure Sequence For One-Rescuer CPR: Adult

1. Establish unresponsiveness. Shake gently and shout, "Are you OK?"
2. Activate EMS system–phone first.
3. Position victim.
4. Establish an airway.

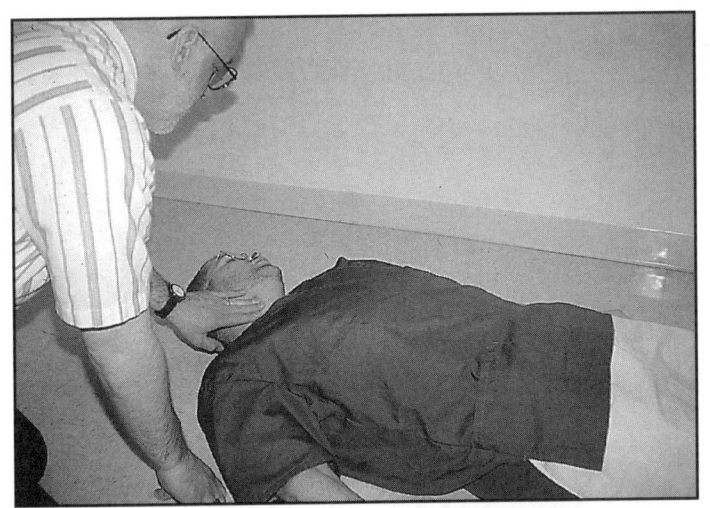

Figure 11-8. Carotid pulse on the adult.

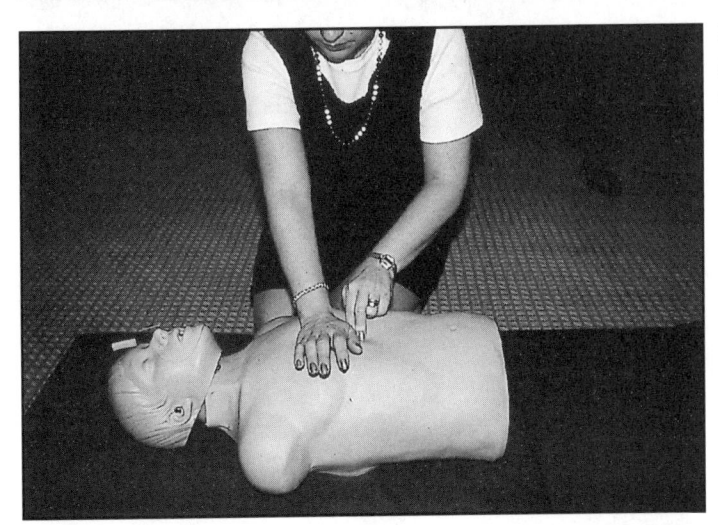

Figure 11-9. Measure two fingers above the xiphoid notch and place one hand on the lower half of the sternum.

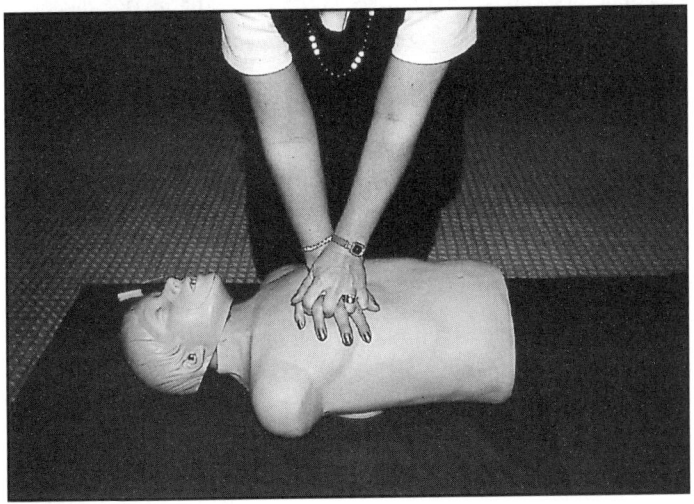

Figure 11-10. Hand position for chest compressions on an adult.

Figure 11-11. The rescuer should lean forward to compress the chest with shoulders directly over the hands.

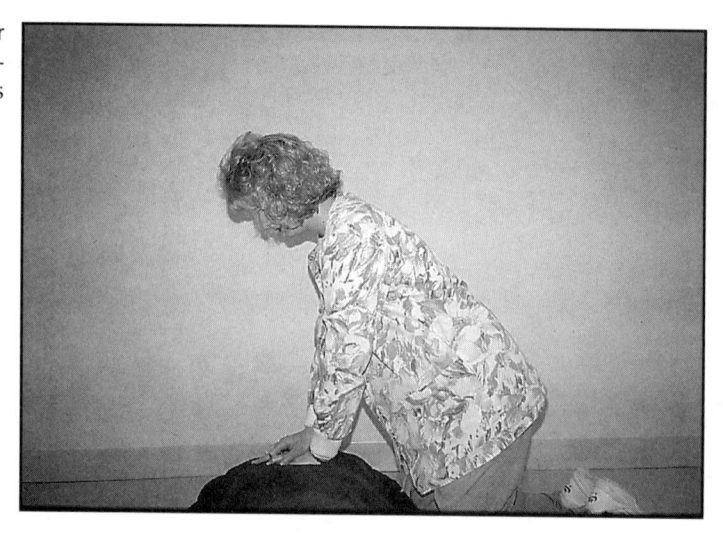

5. Assess breathing. Look, listen, and feel (3 to 5 seconds).
    a. If breathing, place victim in the recovery position and monitor breathing and pulse.
    b. If not breathing:
6. Give 2 slow, full breaths (1.5 to 2 seconds per breath).
7. Assess pulse at carotid artery (5 to 10 seconds).
    a. If there is a pulse, continue rescue breathing at a rate of 1 breath every 5 seconds (approximately 12 breaths per minute).
    b. If there is no pulse:
8. Locate landmarks and position hands over lower half of the sternum.
9. Begin chest compressions counting "one-and-two-and-three-and…" to establish a rhythm. The chest should be depressed 1.5 to 2 inches at a rate of 80 to 100 compressions per minute.
10. Give 15 compressions.
11. Give 2 ventilations.
12. At the end of 4 cycles of 15 compressions and 2 ventilations, check for the return of a pulse.
    a. If there is a pulse but no breathing, rescue breathe at a rate of 1 breath every 5 seconds.
    b. If there is no pulse, resume CPR starting with 2 ventilations followed by chest compressions.
13. Repeat the sequence of 15 compressions and 2 ventilations.
14. Assess for pulse and return of breath every few minutes.

Entrance of Second Layperson Rescuer

The layperson is taught only the one-rescuer CPR technique. If a second rescuer appears and is not identified as a health professional he or she should:
- Identify him or herself
- Ask if EMS has been activated, and call 911 if necessary
- Check for carotid pulse

If there is no pulse, the second rescuer starts one-rescuer CPR and resumes the cycle of 15 compressions to 2 ventilations with as little interruption as possible. When the second rescuer tires, the

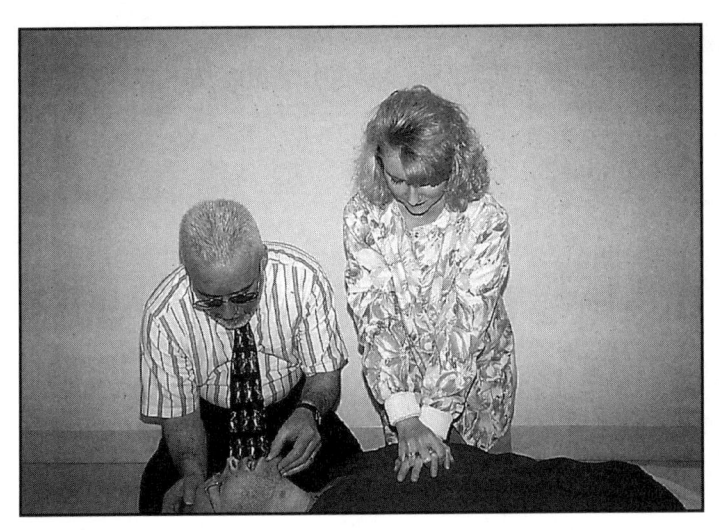

Figure 11-12. Two-rescuer healthcare professional CPR.

two rescuers switch roles and continue monitoring each other's effectiveness of breaths by watching the chest rise during ventilations and feeling for a pulse during compressions.

Procedure Sequence Two-Rescuer CPR (Healthcare Professionals Only): Adult

Notes

Two-rescuer CPR is taught only to healthcare professionals. Two-rescuer CPR is the most efficient way to perform CPR, since it allows compressions and ventilations to be uninterrupted (Figure 11-12). The compression to ventilation ratio is 5:1, with a compression rate of 80 to 100 compressions per minute.

Method

1. Follow procedure for one-rescuer CPR.
2. Second rescuer identifies him or herself by stating "I know CPR, I can help."
3. Asks if EMS system has been activated. If not calls 911.
4. Takes a position on the opposite side of the victim from the first rescuer.
5. First rescuer discontinues compressions. Second rescuer palpates the carotid artery (5 seconds).
    a. If there is no pulse, states "No pulse, resume CPR," and gives a breath.
6. First rescuer resumes compressions at a rate of 80 to 100 per minute, at a ratio of 5 compressions to 1 ventilation.
7. Second rescuer ventilates every 5 compressions and palpates the carotid pulse during chest compressions to evaluate the effectiveness of the compressions.
8. When the first rescuer tires, he or she should call for a switch during counting ("switch-and two-and three-and…").
9. Second rescuer finishes with a ventilation and moves to the chest to find hand positions.

128 Chapter 11

Figure 11-13. Hand position for chest compressions on a child.

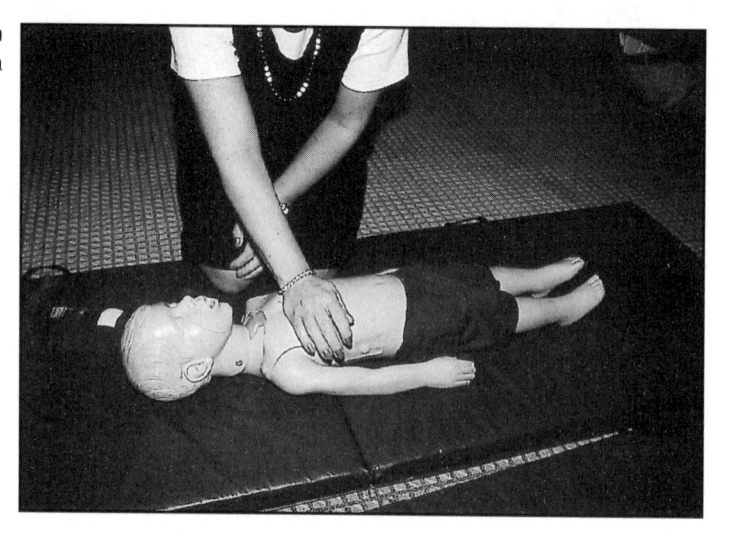

10. First rescuer moves to the head and checks for carotid pulse.
     a. If there is no pulse, states "No pulse, resume CPR," and gives a breath.
11. Repeat compression/ventilation sequence until help arrives.

Procedure Sequence One-Rescuer CPR: Child (1 to 8 years)

Notes

CPR on children ages 1 to 8 is similar to CPR performed on adults with the exception of these four differences:
- If the rescuer is alone, perform 1 minute of CPR before activating the EMS system.
- Use only one hand to perform chest compressions (Figure 11-13).
- Depths of compressions are roughly 1 to 1.5 inches.
- Compress the chest at a slightly faster rate of 100 times per minute, with a ratio of 5 compressions to 1 ventilation.

Method

1. Establish unresponsiveness. Shake gently and shout, "Are you OK?"
2. Call out for help.
3. Position the victim.
4. Establish an airway using head tilt/chin lift method.
5. Assess breathing. Look, listen, and feel.
     a. If breathing, place the victim in the recovery position and monitor breathing and pulse.
     b. If not breathing:
6. Give two slow breaths, 1 to 1.5 seconds per breath.
7. Assess pulse at carotid artery.
     a. If there is a pulse, continue rescue breathing at a rate of 1 breath every 3 seconds and monitor the pulse.
     b. If no pulse:

Cardiopulmonary Resuscitation 129

8. Locate landmarks and position the heel of one hand over the lower sternum.
9. Begin chest compressions at the rate of 80 to 100 compressions per minute and a ratio of 5 compressions to 1 ventilation.
10. After 1 minute of CPR, phone fast for the EMS system (call 911).
11. On returning to the victim, check the carotid pulse.
    a. If there is a pulse, continue rescue breathing at a rate of 1 breath every 3 seconds and monitor the pulse.
    b. If no pulse:
12. Continue the sequence of chest compressions and ventilations.
13. Check for the return of spontaneous breathing and pulse every few minutes until the EMS arrives.

Entrance of Second Rescuer: Child CPR

(Note: Second-rescuer CPR on a child or infant is the same regardless of whether the second rescuer is a layperson or healthcare professional; one person performs CPR at a time, with the second rescuer taking over when the first tires.)

1. Second rescuer identifies him or herself.
2. Asks if EMS has been activated and calls 911 if necessary.
3. First rescuer discontinues compressions. Second rescuer palpates the carotid artery (5 seconds).
    a. If there is a pulse but no breathing, rescue breathe at a rate of 1 breath every 3 seconds.
    b. If there is no pulse:
4. The second rescuer takes over one-rescuer CPR.
5. The first rescuer monitors the second rescuer's ventilations and compressions by watching for the rise and fall of the chest during ventilations and by checking the pulse during compressions.

Procedure Sequence One-Rescuer CPR: Infant (less than 1 year)

Notes

Because of the size of an infant there are several differences in CPR techniques:
- For artificial ventilations, two gentle puffs of air are given covering the infant's nose and mouth (Figure 11-14)
- Check for brachial pulse in the arm (instead of the carotid) (Figure 11-15)
- Hand position for chest compressions is one finger below the imaginary nipple line (Figure 11-16)
- Compressions are given with two fingers at a depth of 0.5 to 1 inch

Method

1. Establish unresponsiveness. Shake gently and shout, "Are you OK?"
2. Call out for help.

Figure 11-14. Artificial ventilations on an infant.

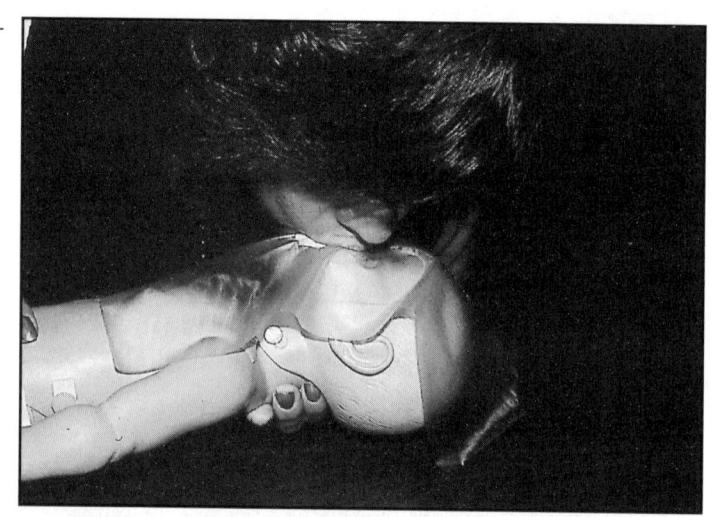

Figure 11-15. Brachial pulse on an infant.

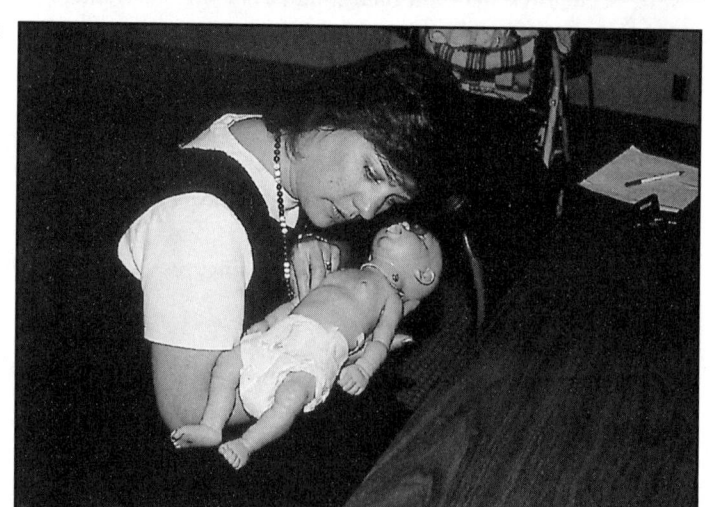

Figure 11-16. Finger position for chest compressions on an infant.

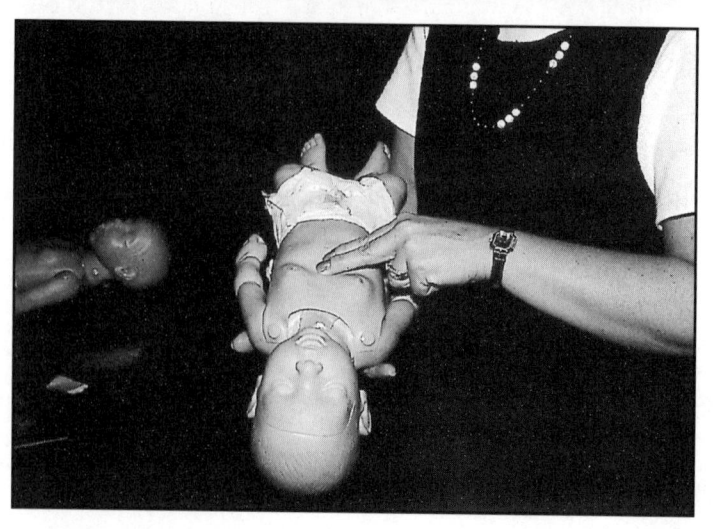

3. Position the victim on his or her back on a firm surface (supporting the head and neck).
4. Establish an airway using head tilt/chin lift method (take care not to hyperextend the neck).
5. Assess breathing. Look, listen, and feel.
    a. If breathing, place the victim in the recovery position maintain an open airway and monitor breathing and pulse.
    b. If not breathing:
6. Give two gentle breaths, covering the nose and mouth (1 to 1.5 seconds per breath).
7. Assess pulse at the brachial artery inside the upper arm.
    a. If there is a pulse, continue rescue breathing at a rate of 1 breath every 3 seconds and monitor the pulse.
    b. If there is no pulse:
8. Locate landmarks by placing two fingers one finger below the imaginary nipple line.
9. Begin chest compressions at a depth of 0.5 to 1 inch per compression, at the rate of 80 to 100 compressions per minute and a ratio of 5 compressions to 1 ventilation.
10. Do 20 cycles of compressions and ventilations (roughly 1 minute of CPR).
11. After 1 minute of CPR, phone fast for the EMS system (call 911).
12. Return to the victim and check the brachial pulse.
    a. If there is a pulse, continue rescue breathing at a rate of 1 breath every 3 seconds and monitor the pulse.
    b. If there is no pulse:
13. Continue sequence chest compressions and ventilations.
14. Check for the return of spontaneous breathing and pulse every few minutes until the EMS arrives.

Obstructed Airway: Adult

It is important to distinguish between a choking victim and other conditions that may appear similar to choking, such as a heart attack or stroke. The universal distress signal for choking is clutching the neck between the thumb and index finger (Figure 11-17).

The victim with a complete airway obstruction is unable to speak or cough. A partial airway obstruction may quickly turn into a situation in which the victim has poor air exchange. A weak, ineffective cough, crowing noises, and cyanosis (blue face) characterize poor air exchange. In either situation, the victim must be treated immediately with the Heimlich maneuver.

Abdominal Thrusts/Heimlich Maneuver

If a person is grasping his or her throat, the rescuer should ask, "Are you choking?" If the victim is unable to speak, perform the Heimlich maneuver. To perform the Heimlich maneuver, stand behind the victim with your legs shoulder width apart. One leg should be slightly in front of the other with your knees slightly bent. This will allow you to catch the victim more easily should he or she fall unconscious. Wrap your arms around the victim's waist and find the point halfway between their xiphoid process and navel (Figure 11-18). Make a fist with your thumb facing towards the victim. With your other hand, grab your fist positioned on the abdomen. Press your fist into the abdomen with quick inward and upward thrusts. Each thrust should be delivered in an attempt to dislodge the FB from the throat of the victim. Continue the abdominal thrusts until the obstruction is dislodged or the victim becomes unconscious.

Figure 11-17. Universal distress signal for choking.

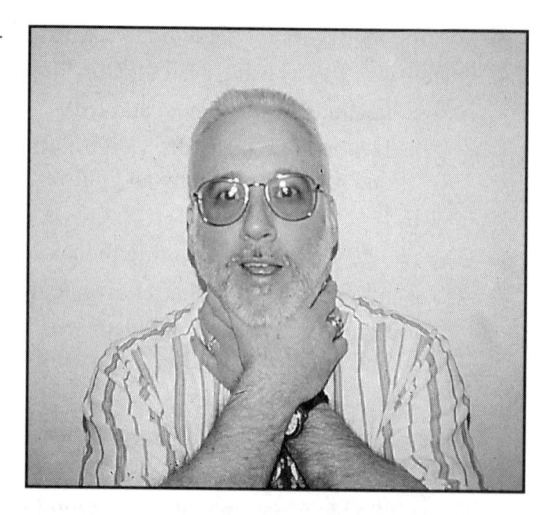

Figure 11-18. Hand position for the Heimlich maneuver on an adult.

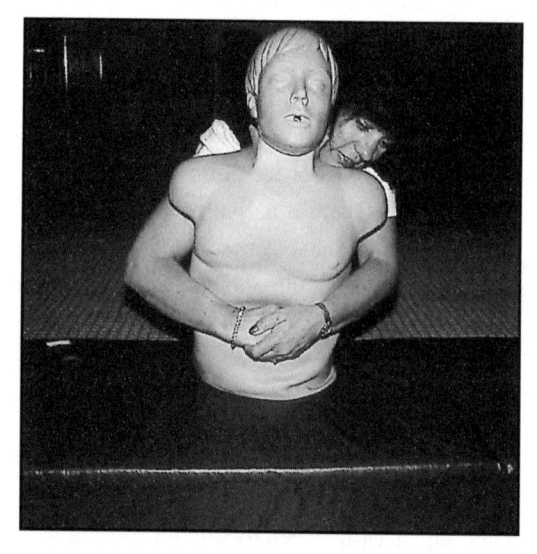

The Heimlich maneuver may also be performed on the victim in the sitting position. Stand behind the victim and place your arms around the chair and the chest of the victim. Locate hand position midway between the navel and the xiphoid process. Deliver the Heimlich maneuver with quick backward thrusts.

If you are unable to wrap your arms around a victim's waist due to pregnancy or obesity, the alternate chest compression method is performed. Wrap your arms under the victim's armpits and around the chest. Position the thumb side of one fist over the lower half of the sternum. Use the other hand to grasp the fist and deliver quick backward chest thrusts. Chest thrusts are continued until the obstruction is dislodged or the victim falls unconscious.

If the obstructed airway is not cleared in a short time, the victim may lose consciousness. If this happens, activate the EMS system by calling 911. Check the victim's mouth for the foreign object by sweeping deeply into their mouth with your hooked index finger (Figure 11-19). Open the airway and attempt to ventilate.

If the breath does not go in, reposition the head and attempt to ventilate a second time. If the airway is still obstructed, perform the Heimlich maneuver by straddling the victim's thighs.

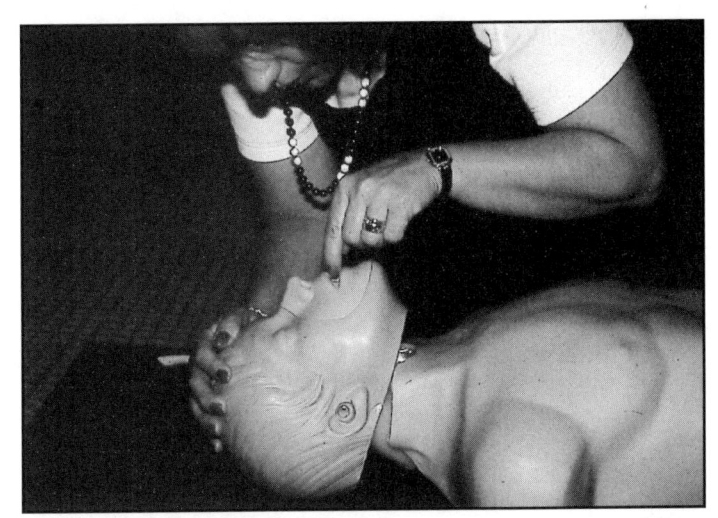

Figure 11-19. Finger sweep on an adult.

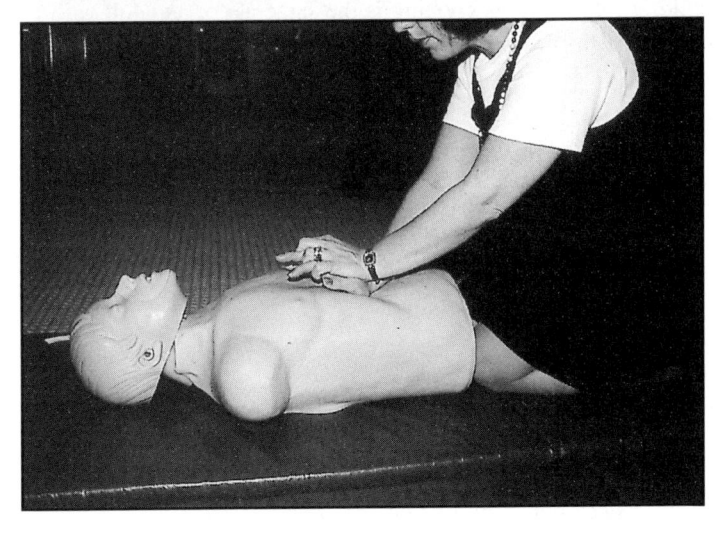

Figure 11-20. Abdominal thrusts on an unconscious adult.

Position the heel of one hand half way between the xiphoid process and the navel. Place the second hand on top of the first and lock fingers together (Figure 11-20). Deliver 5 abdominal thrusts with quick upward movements. Repeat this sequence of finger sweep, ventilations, and abdominal thrusts until the obstruction is removed or help from the EMS arrives.

Procedure Sequence Obstructed Airway: Adult

1. Ask conscious victim, "Are you choking?"
2. Give abdominal thrusts.
3. Repeat thrusts until:
    a. Obstruction is dislodged – monitor breathing.
    b. Victim falls unconscious:
4. Send help to activate the EMS system.
5. Perform tongue/jaw lift. Look in the mouth. Finger sweep.
6. Open airway.
7. Attempt to ventilate:

        a. Ventilation successful – check pulse and monitor breathing.
        b. Ventilation unsuccessful:
    8. Reposition head and attempt to ventilate again.
        a. Ventilation successful – check pulse and monitor breathing.
        b. Ventilation unsuccessful:
    9. Straddle victim's thighs.
    10. Give 5 abdominal thrusts.
    11. Repeat sequence 5 to 10 until:
        a. Obstruction is removed.
        b. EMS arrives.
    12. If airway is not opened after 1 minute, activate the EMS system if not already called.

Obstructed Airway: Child and Infant

The procedure for helping a child or infant who is choking is the same as for an adult with the exception of a blind finger sweep. The finger sweep is done on a child or infant *only* if the obstruction is visible.

Procedure Sequence Obstructed Airway: Child

1. Ask conscious victim, "Are you choking?"
2. Give abdominal thrusts.
3. Repeat thrusts until:
    a. Foreign object is removed – monitor breathing.
    b. Victim falls unconscious:
4. Send help to activate the EMS system.
5. Perform tongue/jaw lift. Look in the mouth. Finger sweep ONLY if obstruction is seen.
6. Open airway.
7. Attempt to ventilate.
    a. Ventilation successful – check pulse and monitor breathing.
    b. Ventilation unsuccessful:
8. Reposition head and attempt to ventilate again.
    a. Ventilation successful – check pulse and monitor breathing.
    b. Ventilation unsuccessful:
9. Straddle victim's thighs.
10. Give 5 abdominal thrusts.
11. Repeat sequence 5 to 10 until:
    a. Foreign object is removed.
    b. EMS arrives.
12. If airway is not opened after 1 minute, activate the EMS system if not already called.

Obstructed Airway: Conscious Infant

The following procedure should be performed on a conscious infant only if a complete airway obstruction is due to a witnessed or suspected foreign object. If the obstruction is caused by swelling due to an infection or reaction, the infant should be rushed to the nearest emergency facility. To begin the procedure for an obstructed airway, place the infant face down over your

Cardiopulmonary Resuscitation 135

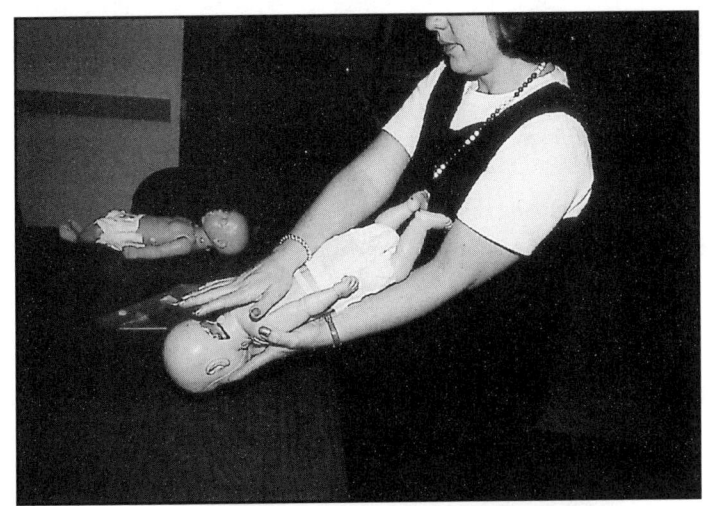

Figure 11-21. Back blows on an infant.

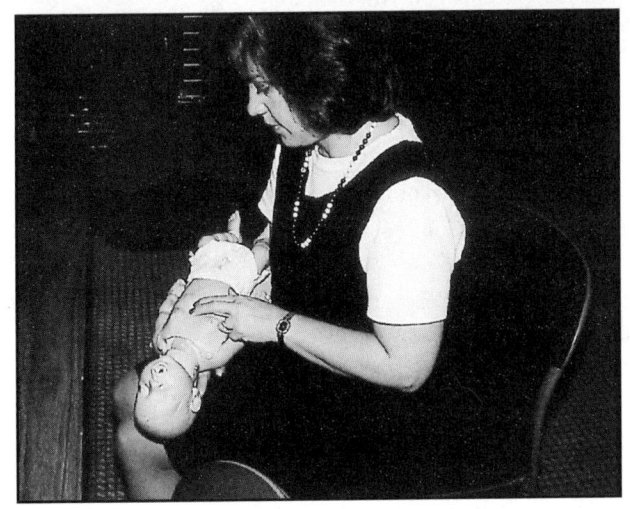

Figure 11-22. Chest thrusts on an infant.

forearm with the head lower than the chest. Support the head by holding your fingers in a "V" on the victim's jaw and resting your forearm on your thigh (Figure 11-21). Deliver 5 back blows between the shoulder blades with the heel of one hand. Again, supporting the head, sandwich the infant between your hands and arms and turn the infant face up. Using the same landmarks as for chest compressions, deliver 5 chest thrusts (Figure 11-22). Each chest thrust should be delivered more slowly than chest compressions and with intent to expel the obstruction. Back blows and chest thrusts should be repeated until either the foreign object is removed or the infant becomes unconscious.

Procedure Sequence Obstructed Airway: Conscious Infant

1. Determine airway obstruction – breathing difficulties, ineffective cough, weak or absent cry, cyanosis (blueness).
2. Place infant face down over arm and deliver 5 back blows.
3. Turn infant face up, supported over arm and deliver 5 chest thrusts.
4. Repeat steps 2 and 3 until:

136 Chapter 11

      a. Foreign object is removed – monitor breathing.
      b. The infant falls unconscious:
5. Call for help.
6. Perform tongue/jaw lift. (Do NOT perform a blind finger sweep. Remove foreign object only if visible.)
7. Attempt to ventilate covering both mouth and nose.
      a. Ventilation successful – monitor breathing.
      b. Ventilation unsuccessful:
8. Reposition head and attempt to ventilate again.
      a. Ventilation successful – monitor breathing.
      b. Ventilation unsuccessful:
9. Deliver 5 back blows.
10. Deliver 5 chest thrusts.
11. Perform tongue/jaw lift and remove foreign object only if visible.
12. Attempt to ventilate.
13. Repeat steps 8 to 12 until successful.
14. If the obstruction is removed check for breathing and pulse.
      a. If breathing, place victim in the recovery position and monitor breathing and pulse.
      b. If not breathing, give 20 rescue breaths per minute and monitor pulse.
      c. If no pulse, give 2 breaths and start cycles of compressions and breaths at a rate of 5:1.
15. If you are alone and your efforts of back blows and chest thrusts are unsuccessful, activate the EMS system after approximately 1 minute of effort to clear the obstruction

Procedure Sequence Obstructed Airway: Unconscious Infant

1. Determine unresponsiveness – tap and shake gently.
2. Call for help.
3. Position the infant.
4. Open the airway (take care not to hyperextend the neck).
5. Determine breathlessness – Look, listen, and feel.
6. Attempt to ventilate covering both mouth and nose.
      a. Ventilation successful – monitor breathing.
      b. Ventilation unsuccessful:
7. Reposition head and attempt to ventilate again, checking the seal over the mouth and nose.
8. Deliver 5 back blows.
9. Deliver 5 chest thrusts.
10. Perform tongue/jaw lift maneuver. Remove object only if seen.
11. Attempt to ventilate.
12. If unsuccessful, reposition and attempt to ventilate again.
13. Repeat steps 8 to 12 until successful.

14. If the obstruction is removed check for breathing and pulse:
    a. If breathing, place victim in the recovery position and monitor breathing and pulse.
    b. If not breathing, give 20 rescue breaths per minute and monitor pulse.
    c. If no pulse, give 2 breaths and start cycles of compressions and breaths at a rate of 5:1.
15. If you are alone and your efforts of back blows and chest thrusts are unsuccessful, activate the EMS system after approximately 1 minute of effort to clear the obstruction.

Bibliography

Albert MA, Jakobiec FA. *Principles and Practice of Ophthalmology, Clinical Practice.* Vol. 1. Philadelphia, Pa: WB Saunders Co; 1994.

Basic Life Support Heartsaver Guide, A Student Handbook for Cardiopulmonary Resuscitation and First Aid for Choking. Dallas, Tex: American Heart Association; 1997.

Benson WE, Shakin J, Sarin LK. Blunt trauma. In: Tasman W, Jaeger EA, eds. *Duane's Ophthalmology on CD-ROM.* Philadelphia, Pa: Lippincott-Raven Publishers; 1996.

Cassin B, Solomon S. *Dictionary of Eye Terminology.* 2nd ed. Gainesville, Fla: Triad Publishing Co; 1990.

Catalano RA. *Ocular Emergencies.* Philadelphia, Pa: WB Saunders, Co; 1992.

Chan CC, Palestine AG, Nussenblatt RB. Sympathetic ophthalmia and Vogt-Koyanagi-Harada syndrome. In: Tasman W, Jaeger EA, eds. *Duane's Ophthalmology on CD-ROM.* Philadelphia, Pa: Lippincott-Raven Publishers; 1996.

Cinotti A. *Handbook of Ophthalmologic Emergencies.* 3rd ed. New York, NY: Elsevier Science Publishing Co, Inc; 1985.

Collins J. *Your Eyes...An Owner's Guide.* Englewood Cliffs, NJ: Prentice Hall; 1995.

Collins MLZ, Nelson LB, Parlato CJ. Ophthalmic and systemic manifestations of child abuse. In: Tasman W, Jaeger EA, eds. *Duane's Ophthalmology on CD-ROM.* Philadelphia, Pa: Lippincott-Raven Publishers; 1996.

Cox MS, Hassen TS. Management for posterior segment trauma. In: Tasman W, Jaeger EA, eds. *Duane's Ophthalmology on CD-ROM.* Philadelphia, Pa: Lippincott-Raven Publishers; 1996.

Crouch ER Jr, Williams PB. Trauma: ruptures and bleeding. In: Tasman W, Jaeger EA, eds. *Duane's Ophthalmology on CD-ROM.* Philadelphia, Pa: Lippincott-Raven Publishers; 1996.

Cullom RD, Chang B. *The Wills Eye Manual, Office and Emergency Room Diagnosis and Treatment of Eye Disease.* 2nd ed. Philadelphia, Pa: JB Lippincott Co; 1994.

For My Patient: Retinal Detachment and Vitreous Surgery. San Francisco, Calif: The Retina Research Fund; 1995.

Forster RK. Endophthalmitis. In: Duane TD, Jaeger EA, eds. *Clinical Ophthalmology.* Vol. 4. Philadelphia, Pa: JB Lippincott Co; 1988.

Gariano R. *Retinal Detachment and Surgical Repair.* Presented at Group Health Cooperative; April 1995; Redmond, Wash.

Gayton JL, Ledford JK. *The Crystal Clear Guide to Sight for Life.* Lancaster, Pa: Starburst Publishers; 1996.

Goldberg S. *Ophthalmology Made Ridiculously Simple.* Miami, Fla: MedMaster Inc; 1991.

Goodin JO. *The Red Eye.* Presented at the annual continuing education program for the Washington Academy of Eye Physicians and Surgeon's Assistants; February 28, 1997; Seattle, Wash.

Hargis L, Parker P. *Triage and Ocular Emergencies.* Presented by Ocular Training Concepts as part of the Ocular Update for Ophthalmic/Optometric Assistants and Nurses; March 1992; Minneapolis, Minn.

Healthcare Professional Guides, Medical Emergencies. Springhouse, Pa: Springhouse Corp; 1998.

Kanski JJ. *Clinical Ophthalmology: A Systematic Approach.* 3rd ed. London, England: Butterworth-Heinemann Ltd; 1994.

Kunz JRM, ed. *The American Medical Association Family Medical Guide.* New York, NY: The Readers Digest Association Inc (by permission of Random House); 1982.

Lindquist TD. *Bacterial and Fungal Keratitis.* Presented at the annual continuing education program for the Washington Academy of Eye Physicians and Surgeon's Assistants; March 13, 1998; Seattle, Wash.

Lutz MH. Clinical types of cataract. In: Tasman W, Jaeger EA, eds. *Duane's Ophthalmology on CD-ROM.* Philadelphia, Pa: Lippincott-Raven Publishers; 1996.

McKillop BR. *Cornea.* Presented at the annual continuing education program for the Washington Academy of Eye Physicians and Surgeon's Assistants; March 1, 1996; Seattle, Wash.

Mead M. *Eye trauma.* Presented at the annual continuing education program of the Joint Commission on Allied Health Personnel in Ophthalmology; November 10, 1998; New Orleans, La.

Murray PI, Fielder AR. *Pocket Book of Ophthalmology.* London, England: Butterworth-Heineman; 1997.

Pau H. *Differential Diagnosis of Eye Diseases.* 2nd revised and enlarged ed. New York, NY; Thieme Medical Publishers, Inc; 1988.

Pavan-Langston D, ed. *Manual of Ocular Diagnosis and Therapy.* 2nd ed. Boston, Mass: Little, Brown and Company; 1985.

Richard JM. *A Manual for the Beginning Ophthalmology Resident.* 3rd ed. Rochester, Minn: American Academy of Ophthalmology; 1980.

Smolin G. Ocular diseases with immunologic properties. In: Tasman W, Jaeger EA, eds. *Duane's Ophthalmology on CD-ROM.* Philadelphia, Pa: Lippincott-Raven Publishers; 1996.

Stamper RL, Wasson PJ. *Ophthalmic Medical Assisting: An Independent Study Course.* 2nd ed. San Francisco, Calif: American Academy of Ophthalmology; 1994.

Stein HA, Slatt BJ, Stein RM. *The Ophthalmic Assistant.* 5th ed. St. Louis, Mo: Mosby; 1988.

Stein HA, Slatt BJ, Stein RM. *The Ophthalmic Assistant.* 6th ed. St. Louis, Mo: Mosby; 1994.

Vaughan DG, Asbury T, Riordan-Eva P. *General Ophthalmology.* 13th ed. Norwalk, Conn: Appleton & Lange; 1992.

Watson P. Diseases of the sclera and episclera. In: Duane TD, Jaeger EA, eds. *Clinical Ophthalmology.* Vol. 4. Philadelphia, Pa: JB Lippincott Co; 1988.

Index

Abrasion, corneal. *See* Corneal abrasion
Acanthamoeba, 33, 35, 36
Acid burns, 6, 16, 37, 97
Acute angle-closure glaucoma, 53, 54, 56
Airway, CPR, 122, 123
Alcohol, chemical burns with, 6, 37
Alkali burns, 5, 6, 16, 37, 60, 97
Allergic conjunctivitis, 88, 90
Allergic reactions, ocular drugs, 111-113
Ammonia, chemical burns with, 5, 6, 16, 37
Anaphylactic shock, 109
Anesthetics, reactions to, 112
Angle-closure glaucoma, 54-57, 64
Anterior uveitis, 57, 64-65, 98-100
Avulsion
    of optic nerve, 81
    of vitreous base, 73

Background diabetic retinopathy (BDR), 75
Bacterial conjunctivitis, 25, 88, 89
Bacterial corneal infiltrates/ulcers, 33, 34, 95, 96
Basal cell carcinoma, eyelid, 15
Battery fluid, chemical burns with, 6, 16
Berlin's edema, 80-81
Beta blockers, reactions to, 112
Bilateral panuveitis, 63, 68
Bleach, chemical burns with, 5, 16
Blepharitis, 13
Blow-out fracture, orbit, 19, 20-21
Blunt trauma
    choroid, 63, 67
    eyelid, 15
    glaucoma and, 58
    hyphema, 57-58, 66-67, 98, 99
    iris, 63, 66
    lens, 46, 60
    macula, 81
    optic nerve, 81
    orbital blow-out fractures, 19, 20-21
    vitreous, 79-81
Branch retinal artery occlusion (BRAO), 78
Branch retinal vein occlusion (BRVO), 78, 79
Breathing, CPR, 122, 124
Broken glasses, 3, 9
Burns, 16, 17. *See* Chemical burns; Radiation burns; Thermal burns

Calcium hydroxide, chemical burns with, 6
Car batteries, acid burns from, 6, 16
Carcinoma, eyelid, 15
Cardiac arrest, 118-120. *See* Cardiopulmonary resuscitation; Emergency cardiac care
Cardiopulmonary resuscitation (CPR), 119-137
    adult, 124-128, 131-133
    child, 128-129, 133-137
    Heimlich maneuver, 131-133
    infant, 129-131, 133-137
    obstructed airway, 131-137
    procedure, 120-137
        airway, 122
        breathing, 122-124
        circulation, 124
        Heimlich maneuver, 131-133
        one-rescuer CPR, 124-127, 128-129
        two-rescuer CPR, 127-128, 129-131
Cataracts, 45, 48-51
Cellulitis. *See* Orbital cellulitis; Preseptal cellulitis
Central retinal artery occlusion (CRAO), 6, 77, 113
Central retinal vein occlusion (CRVO), 6, 77-79, 113
Chalazion, 9, 12-13
Chalcosis, 51, 82
Chemical burns, 5, 6
    conjunctiva, 36, 38
    cornea, 25, 37-38
    emergency treatment, 114-115
    eyelid, 11, 16-17
    keratitis, 97
    secondary glaucoma and, 60
Choroid
    anatomy, 64
    hemorrhages, 67
    prolapse, 63, 67
    rupture, 81
    trauma, 63, 67, 81
Cicatricial ectropion, 17
Ciliary body, anatomy, 64
Ciliary flush, 100
Circulation, CPR, 124
Cleaning fluid, chemical burns with, 6, 37
Colored halos, 8

Commotio retinae, 80-81
Conjunctiva
    anatomy, 12, 25, 26
    infections and inflammations, 25, 26-27, 88-90
    pinguecula, 90, 91
    pterygium, 90, 92
    subconjunctival hemorrhage, 90, 91
    trauma
        chemical burn, 36, 38
        foreign body, 39
        lacerations, 43
Conjunctivitis, 25, 26-27, 88, 89
    allergic, 88, 90
    bacterial, 25, 88, 89
    differential diagnosis, 64
    giant papillary conjunctivitis, 35
    gonococcal, 25, 26
    keratoconjunctivitis sicca, 90, 91
    mucopurulent, 26, 27, 89
    neonatal, 88
    viral, 25, 88, 89
Contact lens wearers
    acanthamoeba infection, 33, 35, 36
    corneal abrasions, 35
    giant papillary conjunctivitis, 35
    keratitis/ulcers, 35, 97
    pain or redness, 7
Copper foreign body, 51, 82
Cornea, 93
    anatomy, 25, 29-30, 93-94
    infections and inflammations, 25, 30-36
        corneal graft rejection, 35, 36
        erosion, 30-31, 94-95
        infiltrates, 31, 33, 34
        keratitis, 31-35
        ulcers, 31-34, 95, 96
    trauma
        abrasion, 7, 39, 40, 94
        burns, 25, 37-39
        foreign bodies, 25, 39-41, 42
        lacerations, 25, 41-43
    urgent conditions, 30-35
Corneal graft rejection, 35, 36
"Crash cart," 105, 106
Cryotherapy, 74, 75

Cystoid macular edema, 76

Defibrillation, 120
Detached retina. *See* Retinal detachment
Diabetes
    insulin shock, 109-110
    retinopathy, 75
Discharge, 9
Distorted vision, 8
Double vision, 8
Drain cleaner, chemical burns with, 5, 16, 37
Droopy lid, 8
Drug reactions, emergency treatment, 111-113
Dry eye, 90, 91

Ectopia lentis, 46
Ectropion, 13-14, 17, 87
Electromagnetic radiation, cataracts, 51
Emergency cardiac care (ECC), 117, 118
    advanced cardiac life support (ACLS), 118, 120
    cardiopulmonary resuscitation, 119-131
    chain of survival, 119
    emergency medical services, 119
Emergency cart, 105, 106
Emergency medical system (EMS), 105, 106, 119
Emergency treatment
    assessment, 106-107
    cardiac emergencies. *See* Emergency cardiac care
    cardiopulmonary resuscitation, 119-131
    "crash cart," 105, 106
    drug reactions, 111-113
    emergency response team, 105, 109, 117-119
    eye pain, 114
    obstructed airway, 131-137
    ocular emergencies, 5-7, 113-115
    office preparation for, 106
    triage. *See* Triage
    when doctor is out, 115
Endophthalmitis, 83, 101
Entropion, 13-14, 87
Episcleritis, 28-29, 93, 94
Epithelial ingrowth, glaucoma and, 58
Erosion, corneal. *See* Corneal erosion

External hordeolum, 9, 12
Eyeglasses, broken, 3, 9
Eyelid, 11
    abnormalities
        ectropion, 13-14, 17, 87
        entropion, 13-14, 87
        trichiasis, 14, 87-88
    anatomy, 12
    infections and inflammations, 11, 12-13, 86
    lesions, 9
    malignant tumors, 11, 14-15
    trauma, 7
        blunt trauma, 15
        burns, 11, 16-17
        lacerations, 11, 16
Eye pain, 7, 8, 114
Eye redness, 86-102
    anterior chamber, 98
    conjunctiva, 88-92
    contact lens wearers, 7
    cornea, 93-97
    differential diagnosis, 101
    for more than 3 weeks, 9
    ocular adnexa, 86-88
    patient history, 101-102
    sclera, 92-93
    uveal tract, 98-100

Fainting, emergency treatment, 108
Falls, emergency treatment, 110-111
First aid. *See* Emergency cardiac care; Emergency treatment; Triage
Floaters, 7, 74
Fluorescein dyes, reactions to, 112
Foreign bodies (FB), 7, 51
    conjunctiva, 39
    cornea, 25, 39-41, 42
    metallic, 51, 82
    nonmetallic, 82
    orbit, 19, 21-22
    vitreous, 82
Fovea, 72
Fractures, orbital blow-out fractures, 19, 20-21
Fungal keratitis, 33, 34

Gasoline, chemical burns with, 6, 37

Ghost cell glaucoma, 58
Giant papillary conjunctivitis, 35
Glassblower's cataract, 51
Glasses, broken, 3, 9
Glaucoma
    defined, 54
    ghost cell glaucoma, 58
    hemolytic glaucoma, 57-58
    lens particle glaucoma, 59
    neovascular glaucoma, 59
    phacolytic glaucoma, 59
    phacomorphic glaucoma, 59
    primary glaucoma, 53, 54
        primary angle-closure glaucoma (PACG), 54-57, 64, 98
        primary open-angle glaucoma (POAG), 54, 55
    secondary glaucoma, 53, 57, 65
        chemical burns, 60
        lens-related, 59-60
        obstructed trabeculum, 57-59
    uveitis and, 57
Gonococcal conjunctivitis, 25, 26

Headaches, 9
Heimlich maneuver, 131-133
Hemolytic glaucoma, 57-58
Hemorrhage. *See also* Hyphema
    choroidal, 67
    retinal, 75-77
    subconjunctival, 90, 91
    vitreous, 6, 73, 74, 75, 80
Herpes simplex virus, keratitis, 31-32, 95
Herpes zoster virus, keratitis, 32-33, 34, 96
Histoplasmosis, uveitis associated with, 100
Hordeolum, 9, 12
Hypermature cataract, 49
Hyphema, 57-58, 66-67, 98, 99

Immature cataract, 49, 50
Infants
    emergency treatment
        CPR, 129-131
        obstructed airway, 133-137
    neonatal conjunctivitis, 88
    shaken baby syndrome, 83

Infections and inflammations
    conjunctiva, 25, 26-27, 35, 88-90
    contact lens wearers, 35, 97
    cornea, 25, 30-36, 95-97
    eyelid, 11, 12-13, 86
    hypopyon, 98, 99
    iris, 63, 64-66, 98-100
    orbit, 19, 22, 86-87
    sclera, 25, 27-29, 92-93
    uvea, 63, 64-66, 98-100
    vitreous, 83
Infiltrates, corneal. *See* Corneal infiltrates
Insulin shock, emergency treatment, 109-110
Internal hordeolum, 12
Intraocular lens (IOL) implant, 48
Intraorbital foreign bodies, 19, 21-22
Intumescent cataract, 49
Iridodialysis, 66
Iridodonesis, 46, 66
Iridotomy, 57
Iris
    anatomy, 64
    blunt trauma, 63, 66
    infections and inflammations, uveitis, 63,
        64-66, 98-100
    iridodonesis, 46, 66
Iritis, 64-65, 66, 98-100
Iron foreign body, 51, 82
Itching, 9

Keratitic precipitates, 65
Keratitis, 31-35, 95-97
    fungal, 33, 34
    ocular herpes, 31-33, 34, 95
    superficial punctate keratitis (SPK), 38
Keratoconjunctivitis sicca, 90, 91
Kerosene, chemical burns with, 6, 37

Lacerations
    choroidal prolapse, 63, 67
    conjunctiva, 43
    cornea, 25, 41-43
    eyelid, 11, 16
Lacrimal system
    anatomy, 12
    infections and inflammations, 86-87

Lens
    anatomy, 45, 46, 47
    cataracts, 45, 48-51
    secondary glaucoma, 59-60
    trauma, 49
        dislocation, 46-48, 60, 66
Lens particle glaucoma, 59
Lenticular dislocation, 46-48, 60, 66
Lids. *See* Eyelid
Light sensitivity, 8
Lime, chemical burns with, 6
Loss of vision. *See* Visual loss
Luxation, lens, 46

Macula, 72
    edema, 76, 77, 81
    holes, 75, 76
Macular degeneration, 75, 77
Malignant tumors, eyelid, 11, 14-15
Mature cataract, 49, 50
Metallic foreign body, 51, 82
Morgagnian cataract, 49
Mucopurulent conjunctivitis, 26, 27, 89

Nasolacrimal duct obstruction, 13
Neonatal conjunctivitis, 88
Neovascular glaucoma, 59

Obstructed airway, emergency treatment, 131-137
Ocular adnexa, 86-88
Ocular drugs, allergic reactions, 111-113
Ocular emergencies, 5-7. *See also* Triage
    procedures, 113-115
    treatment within hours, 7
    treatment within minutes, 6-7
Ocular herpes, 31-33, 34, 95
Ocular histoplasmosis, uveitis associated with,
    100
Ocular trauma
    blunt trauma. *See* Blunt trauma
    chemical burns. *See* Chemical burns
    choroid, 63, 67, 81
    conjunctiva, 36, 38, 39, 43
    cornea, 7, 25, 37-39, 41-43
    emergency treatment, 114
    external globe trauma, 35, 37-43

eyelid, 7, 11, 15-17
foreign bodies. *See* Foreign bodies
glaucoma and, 58
hyphema, 57-58, 66-67, 98, 99
iris, 63, 66
lacerations. *See* Lacerations
lens, 46, 47, 49-51, 60
macula, 81
optic nerve, 81
orbit, 19, 20-22
penetrating injury. *See* Penetrating injury
posterior segment, 79-83
retina, 6, 71, 74-75, 80, 82
shaken baby syndrome, 83
thermal burns. *See* Thermal burns
vitreous, 79-83
Open-angle glaucoma, 54, 55
Optic nerve injuries, 81
Orbit, 19
anatomy, 20, 21
infections and inflammation, 12, 19, 22, 86-87
trauma
blow-out fractures, 19, 20-21
foreign bodies, 19, 21-22
Orbital cellulitis, 12, 19, 22, 86
Organic solvents, chemical burns with, 6, 36
Oven cleaner, chemical burns with, 16, 37

Pachymetry, 30
Papilledema, 81
Paracentesis, 113
Pars planitis, uveitis associated with, 100
Penetrating injury, 7
sympathetic ophthalmia, 63, 67-68
vitreous, 81-82
Penicillins, reactions to, 112
Phacodonesis, 46
Phacolytic glaucoma, 59
Phacomorphic glaucoma, 59
Photophobia, 8
Pinguecula, 90, 92
"Pink eye". *See* Conjunctivitis
Pneumatic retinopexy, 74
Posterior uveitis, 65-66, 100
Preseptal cellulitis, 12, 87

Primary glaucoma, 53, 54
primary angle-closure glaucoma (PACG), 54-57, 64, 98
primary open-angle glaucoma (POAG), 54, 55
Proliferative diabetic retinopathy (PDR), 75
Pterygium, 90, 92
Ptosis, 8
Purtscher's retinopathy, 82

Radiation burns, 38-39, 51
Recurrent corneal erosion, 30-31, 94-95
Redness. *See* Eye redness
Retina
anatomy, 71, 72, 73
Berlin's edema, 80-81
commotio retinae, 80-81
detached, 6, 71, 74-75, 80
hemorrhage, 75-77
tears, 74
trauma
detachment, 6, 71, 74-75, 80
Purtscher's retinopathy, 82
shaken baby syndrome, 83
Retinopathy
diabetic, 75
Purtscher's retinopathy, 82
Rupture of the globe, 81

Sarcoidosis, uveitis associated with, 100
Sclera
anatomy, 25, 27
choroidal prolapse, 63, 67
infections and inflammations, 25, 27-29, 92-94
Scleral buckle, 74
Scleritis, 25, 27-28, 92-93
Sebaceous gland carcinoma, 15
Secondary glaucoma, 53, 57-60, 65
Seidel's test, 39, 41
Seizures, emergency treatment, 110
Shaken baby syndrome, 83
Shingles, 32, 96
Shock, emergency treatment, 108-109
Siderosis, 51, 82
Soft contact lens wearers, 35, 97

Squamous cell carcinoma, eyelid, 15
Steroids, reactions to, 112
Stye, 9, 12
Subconjunctival hemorrhage, 90, 91
Subluxation, lens, 47-48
Sulfa drugs, reactions to, 111-112
Superficial punctate keratitis (SPK), 38
Sympathetic ophthalmia, 63, 67-68
Syphilis, uveitis associated with, 100

Thermal burns, cornea, 38
Toilet cleaner, chemical burns with, 5
Total dislocation of the lens, 46
Toxoplasmosis, uveitis associated with, 100
Trauma. *See* Ocular trauma
Traumatic angle recession, 58
Traumatic cataracts, 49-51
Traumatic detachment, 80
Traumatic iritis, 66
Triage, 1-9
    cardiac emergencies, 119-131
    elective category, 8-9
    emergent conditions, 5-7
    general medical emergencies, 106-113
    ocular emergencies, 113-115
    office triage, 2-3
    patient history, 3-5, 101-102
    screening, 2-5
    telephone calls, 2
    urgent category, 8, 12, 30-35
    when doctor is out, 115
Trichiasis, 14, 87-88
Tumors, eyelid, 11, 14-15

Ulcers, corneal. *See* Corneal ulcers
Ultraviolet light, keratitis, 97
Uvea
    anatomy, 63, 64, 98
    infections and inflammations, 63, 64-66, 98-100
Uveitis, 63, 64-66
    anterior uveitis, 57, 64-65, 98-99
    bilateral panuveitis, 63, 68
    glaucoma and, 57
    posterior uveitis, 65-66, 100

Vascular occlusions, 77-79
Viral conjunctivitis, 25, 88, 89
Visual loss
    gradual, 9
    sudden and painless, 6, 113
Vitrectomy, 74
Vitreous
    anatomy, 72, 100
    endophthalmitis, 83, 101
    floaters, 7, 74
    hemorrhage, 6, 73, 74, 75, 80
    posterior vitreous detachment, 72
    trauma
        blunt trauma, 79-81
        foreign bodies, 82
        penetrating and perforating injuries, 81-82
    vascular occlusions, 77-79
Vossius' ring, 66

Wet macular degeneration, 75, 77

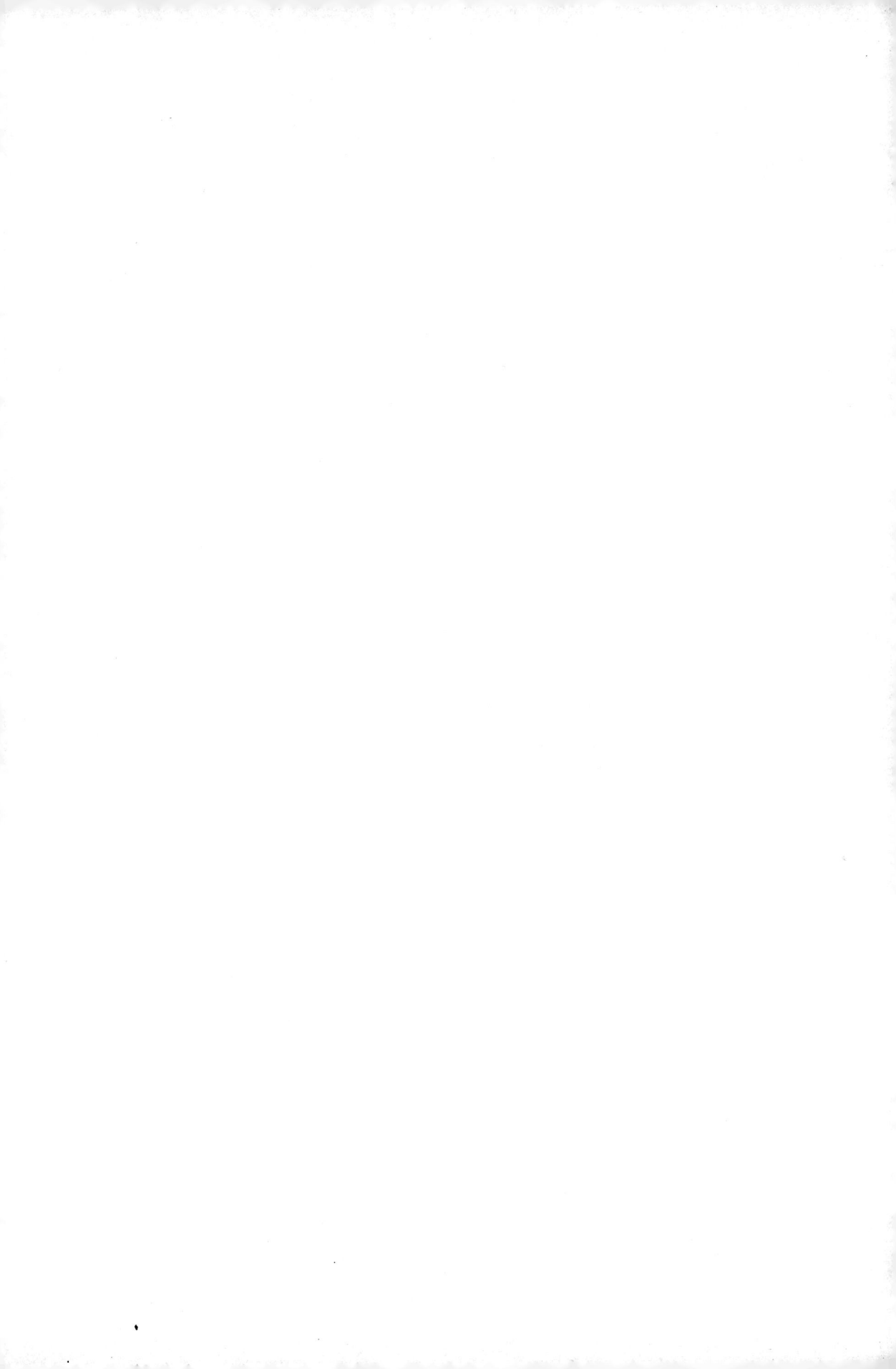

The Basic Bookshelf for Eyecare Professionals

Encourage education, refine office knowledge, and increase office efficiency with *The Basic Bookshelf for Eyecare Professionals series*.

Title	Author	Book#	Price
☐ Basic Procedures	DuBois	63470	$30.00
☐ Cataract and Glaucoma	Duvall	63357	$24.00
☐ COA Exam Review Manual	Ledford	63330	$33.00
☐ COMT Exam Review Manual	Ledford	64221	$33.00
☐ COT Exam Review Manual	Ledford	63241	$33.00
☐ Clinical Ocular Photography	Cunningham	63772	$30.00
☐ Contact Lenses	Daniels	63454	$30.00
☐ Emergencies in Eyecare	Hargis	63543	$30.00
☐ Frames and Lenses	Carlton	63640	$30.00
☐ General Medical Knowledge	Bittinger	63349	$30.00
☐ Instrumentation for Eyecare Paraprofessionals	Herrin	63993	$30.00
☐ Low Vision Handbook, The	Brown	63292	$30.00
☐ Ocular Anatomy and Physiology	Lens	63489	$30.00
☐ Office and Career Management	Borover	63314	$30.00
☐ Ophthalmic Medications and Pharmacology	Duvall	63284	$26.00
☐ Ophthalmic Surgical Assistant, The	Boess-Lott	64035	$30.00
☐ Optics, Retinoscopy, and Refractometry	Lens	63977	$30.00
☐ Overview of Ocular Disorders	Gwin	63365	$30.00
☐ Overview of Ocular Surgery and Surgical Counseling	Pickett	63322	$30.00
☐ Quick Reference Glossary, 2E	Hoffman	63705	$22.00
☐ Refractive Surgery for Eyecare Paraprofessionals	Gayton	63373	$21.00
☐ Slit Lamp Primer, The	Ledford	63306	$30.00
☐ Special Skills and Techniques	Van Boemel	63497	$30.00
☐ Systematic Approach to Strabismus, A	Hansen	63268	$27.00
☐ Visual Fields	Choplin	63632	$33.00

Subtotal $_____
NJ residents add 6% sales tax $_____
Handling Charge $ **4.50**
Total $_____

ORDER TODAY!

Name: _____
Address: _____
City: _____ State: _____ Zip Code: _____
Phone: _____ Fax: _____

Charge my: ___American Express ___Visa ___Mastercard Account#: _____
Exp. date: _____ Signature: _____

Prices are subject to change. Shipping charges may apply.

Mail order form to:
SLACK Incorporated, Professional Book Division, 6900 Grove Road, Thorofare, NJ 08086-9447
Call: (800) 257-8290, (609) 848-1000, or (856) 848-1000 • Fax: (609) 853-5991 or (856) 853-5991
Send an email to orders@slackinc.com • Visit our World Wide Web site at www.slackinc.com

CODE: 6A416

For your information

This book and many others on numerous different topics are available from SLACK Incorporated. For further information or a copy of our latest catalog, contact us at:

> *Professional Book Division*
> *SLACK Incorporated*
> *6900 Grove Road*
> *Thorofare, NJ 08086 USA*
> *Telephone: 1-609-848-1000*
> *1-800-257-8290*
> *Fax: 1-609-853-5991*
> *E-mail: orders@slackinc.com*
> *WWW: http://www.slackinc.com*

We accept most major credit cards and checks or money orders in US dollars drawn on a US bank. Most orders are shipped within 72 hours.

Contact us for information on recent releases, forthcoming titles, and bestsellers. If you have a comment about this title or see a need for a new book, direct your correspondence to the Editorial Director at the above address.

*If you are an instructor, we can be reached at the address listed above or on the Internet at **educomps@slackinc.com** for specific needs.*

Thank you for your interest and we hope you found this work beneficial.